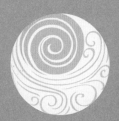

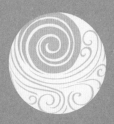

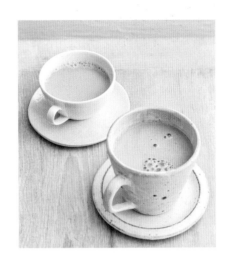

the self-healing
REVOLUTION

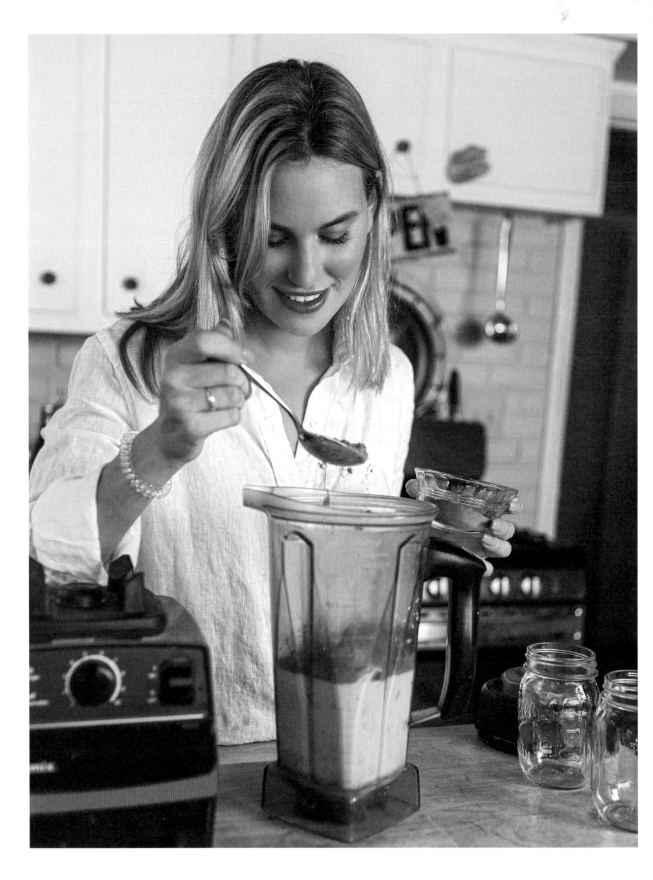

the self-healing REVOLUTION

modern-day **Ayurveda**

with recipes and tools for intuitive living

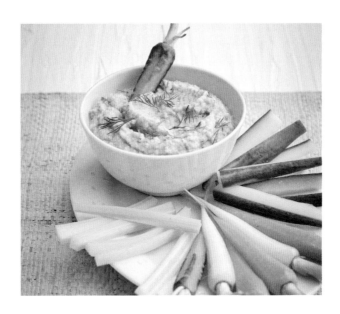

NOELLE RENÉE KOVARY

CICO BOOKS

LONDON NEW YORK

To my best friend and guardian angel, Jacklyn Michelle Henderson, through your life and death you've given me the courage to believe in my power to heal. This one's for you.

Published in 2019 by CICO Books
An imprint of Ryland Peters & Small Ltd
20–21 Jockey's Fields   341 E 116th St
London WC1R 4BW   New York, NY 10029

www.rylandpeters.com

10 9 8 7 6 5 4 3 2 1

ISBN: 978-1-78249-697-7

Printed in China

Editor: Clare Churly
Designer: Emily Breen
Illustrators: Cathy Brear, Stephen Dew, and Anthony Duke
Recipe photographer: Stephen Conroy
Stylist: Kim Sullivan
Home economist: Kate Wesson
For additional photography credits, see page 160.

Commissioning editor: Kristine Pidkameny
Senior editor: Carmel Edmonds
Art director: Sally Powell
Production manager: Gordana Simakovic
Publishing manager: Penny Craig
Publisher: Cindy Richards

NOTES
Both American (Imperial plus US cups) and British (Metric) measurements are included in these recipes for convenience; however, it is important to work with one set of measurements and not alternate between the two within a recipe.

The views expressed in this book are those of the author, but they are general views only, and readers are urged to consult a relevant and qualified specialist or physician for individual advice before beginning any dietary regimen.

Contents

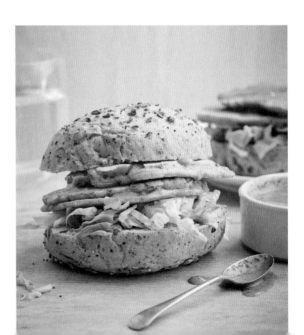

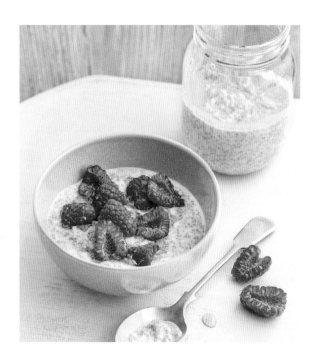

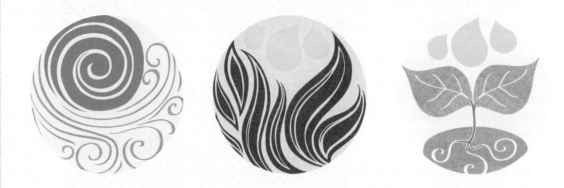

You are the creator of your dreams, and the master of your life. Honor your journey and don't rush to the end; the middle is where you will find your strength. Focus on the moment right in front of you, and see how you can turn an obstacle into a masterpiece.

Introduction

Are you searching for a better body, a more resilient mind, and overall longevity? If the answer is yes, this book will introduce you to age-old practices that can increase vitality, balance, resilience, and happiness. With this book as your guide, you will master the tools you need to own the power you have to heal your life and live in your most balanced state.

The information in this book is for everyone. It is for you, your friends, your mother, your lover, and anyone who needs to gain the knowledge of self-healing. I hope you will pass on the knowledge you gain from this book to other people with the intent of educating and helping them. I hope the topics I cover here are spoken about around your dinner table, in the lunchroom, at bars with your friends, at soccer practice, and in all the places where people meet and discovery starts.

Just like you, I was once on a quest to heal my body and desperate for guidance. I'm one in a million. I'm special and rare. But it's not what you think. I'm a contradiction in terms. Of course, to be a healer, an empath, an alchemist, and even a good witch doctor (all names I've been labeled) is rare and very special but it's why (and how) I am those things that has shaped my story. My experiences have led me to become passionate about teaching and educating others with the tools that have been integral and invaluable in the process of my own healing … because, you see, I was my own first patient.

When I was fourteen, my life was the typical teenage affair of carefree days filled with the activities of a vibrant, healthy, sporty, curious, fun-loving, sensitive, creative, and spirited young person until I began to experience debilitating symptoms that slowly and steadily turned my life into a blur of hopelessness. After nearly three years of consulting an endless parade of medical experts, including nephrologists, gynecologists, dermatologists, and psychologists, I was eventually diagnosed with Gitleman syndrome, a rare incurable kidney disorder that statistically, you guessed it, affects one in a million people.

As it turned out, the diagnosis was just the beginning of my journey. I was soon to discover that the Western doctors whose care I was under were not that interested in helping me to find ways to alleviate the side effects from the massive amounts of meds I needed to take in order to survive. I was at a crossroads of despair and futility.

It was this moment that I realized I was in a do-or-die situation. I knew I had to take control of my life by finding ways to alleviate the pain I was experiencing—both physically and mentally. Intuitively, my interest in nutrition and exercise became the first stepping-stone in my search for alternative ways to improve the quality of my life. My quest eventually led me to the realms of Eastern medicine, where I discovered the concepts of self-love and self-care that I now know can benefit those people who seek ways to improve their lives. Twelve years after the first symptoms of a rare disease began to ravage my body and spirit, I have established a self-care routine and significantly healed my body, mind, and spirit. For me, however, this is an ongoing voyage of discovery; it is a lifelong journey.

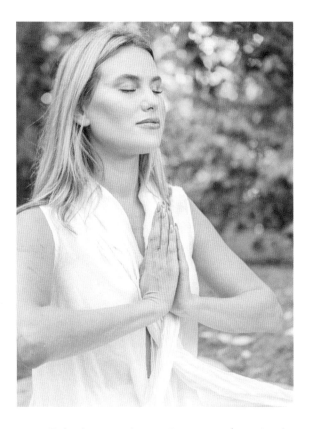

Today, I am proud to practice as a transformational mentor, certified Ayurvedic counselor, Reiki healer, herbalist, alchemist, and–yes–a good witch doctor who is hell bent on healing the imbalance in people's lives. I enjoy good music, fine food, cooking, making chocolate, traveling to foreign lands, the ocean, a great book, the purr of a cat, the sound of rain, the feel of the sun on my face, a warm bath, an excellent tonic, dancing, intimate conversations, informed debate, a good laugh, and hugs.

My journey has inspired me to share the deep wisdom Ayurveda (and beyond) has brought me. I want to pass this knowledge on to help others because I know what it's like to feel lost, confused, and constantly searching for peace and balance. I wrote this book because I wish I had found a book like this to guide me at the start of my quest. I wish someone had been able to hand me a book that would have helped me heal myself without the torment of jumping through hoops and sacrificing so much of my happiness along the way.

Even if you're not suffering from a chronic illness, the tools in this book are necessary for life. We all have physical and emotional pain that we experience in different ways on different days. If I didn't have these tools, I wouldn't be able to get through my traumas with the sincerity of positivity that I do.

I want this book to be your permanent guide– something to fall back on when you need to find yourself or when you aren't getting what you need from the external world. I want to teach you why this kind of deep self-love and respect is so important. I want to show you how to navigate life with simplicity and ease. I want to pass on this knowledge in the most appetizing and inspiring way possible. Everyone has the right to know they already have the power to heal themselves.

Thank you for joining me here and sharing in my journey. Thank you for choosing self-love. Thank you for taking action.

So What is Ayurveda?

Ayurveda is a 5,000-year-old, tried-and-true medicinal system that uses simple daily practices, herbs, and nutrition to bring the body and mind to a state of balance and well-being. The word Ayurveda means "the science of life." In Ayurveda, we consider and look at not only the body but also the mind and lifestyle of an individual. We believe that Ayurveda can help to uncover and decode the mysteries behind health and healing and that the true secret to living in balance is already inside us. Combining spiritual, psychological, and physiological science, Ayurveda sees each individual as a unique creation of the universe. This methodology encompasses specific practices, recipes, guidelines, and remedies to balance the energy systems that flow throughout each individual. The beauty of Ayurveda is that it is a system that anyone can follow. From the simplest tools, like drinking warm water with lemon before a meal, to more complex solutions, such as making home remedies to treat indigestion, this book covers it all.

The practice of Ayurveda will deepen your understanding of self and what it means to create light out of dark. Often times, our "mess" is actually our message. Ayurveda helps to peel away the layers to expose the truth behind our "mess." Within this book you will find age-old tools to heal your body, mind, and spirit–and you can do this without even giving up your weekly glass of red wine or square of dark chocolate. The premise behind Ayurveda is to be in tune with your true nature as well as the environment that surrounds you. Finding your own specific balance will help you live a life full of health and happiness. The journey to find your true nature requires you to get really honest with yourself and bring consciousness to every part of your body and life. It also means coming to the realization that everything you do, from the time you wake up in the morning to the time you go to sleep at night has an effect on the balance of your body and mind.

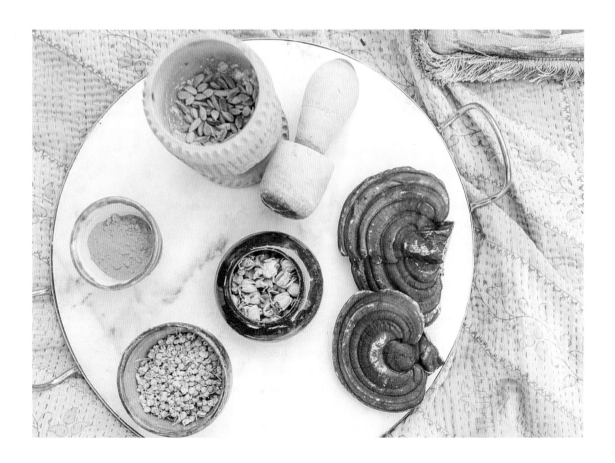

A New Lifestyle

Ditch the diet dogmas and start living your best life, all day every day. The advice in this book is not a fad you will follow and then fall away from. It is paradigm shift in a world obsessed with diets and quick fixes. This is your life and you deserve to be in control of it. This book will provide you with the power of knowledge. You will learn to simplify your life, establish rituals, and explore the alchemist within you to make sound and positive choices throughout all areas of your daily life. You will learn to be gentle and kind through all phases of transformation. As you use these tools to heal your life, slowly you will begin to make permanent and positive transitions.

There is a fine line between doing the right amount of due diligence for your health and obsessing over it. Counting every calorie you eat will not help you to sustain a healthy figure. Labeling yourself by the food you eat will not grant you freedom around food. Depriving yourself of pleasure will not mean you are healthy. In order to heal, you must leave room for change and acceptance, which are integral to the process of transformation. Understanding your specific nature and your unique balance will help ease some of your reservations about letting go of these restrictions and old patterns. You will begin to see why this is a lifestyle, not a diet.

Diets are temporary, they restrict our needs (physically and emotionally), and create road blocks that often lead us back to square one. The truth is, you can't fake healing, which is why this is a lifestyle book and not a kitschy diet program to help you lose ten pounds in three weeks before your best friend's wedding. Healing takes time, effort, and consistency. Whether you are experiencing a mild case of indigestion and bloating or struggling with a long-term illness, consistency and dedication to yourself is key. Healing is not linear, you may take two steps forward, then three steps backward, and then another step to the side. That is true healing in the works. That is okay.

Throwing away your time limit or "finish-line goals" is essential in making this process work for you. When we set ourselves up against a force beyond our control (unrealistic goals), we set ourselves up for a letdown. We are not the keepers of time and we are not in control of how long it will take for a body to heal and change. We are dealing with sensitive and real energy here. There are no quick fixes. So let go of thoughts such as "next year I won't be sick anymore," "I have to reach my peak performance or I'm not good enough," "I need to be skinny by summer," "it's been six months and I haven't gained any muscle," "if my skin doesn't clear by next week I'll quit," or "I haven't lost any weight and I've been dieting for a month." The moment you drop these thought patterns and time lines, and the pressure to set goals, healing gets easier and progress happens.

You are in control of everything you put in your body. You are in control of the environments you live and work in, your thoughts, your actions, and your desire to improve. Take control of what you have and stop focusing on all the things you think you don't have. Ayurveda is not a quick fix or the next fad, it is ancient system of healing that will provide long-term wellness and longevity for those who wish to do the work.

This new lifestyle is not just about weight loss or physical changes, it is the beginning of truly knowing yourself. Of course, you will lose weight (or gain weight) if that's what you need; you will increase your energy levels; you will become stronger in body and mind; you will improve your digestion, teeth, hair, and skin; and you

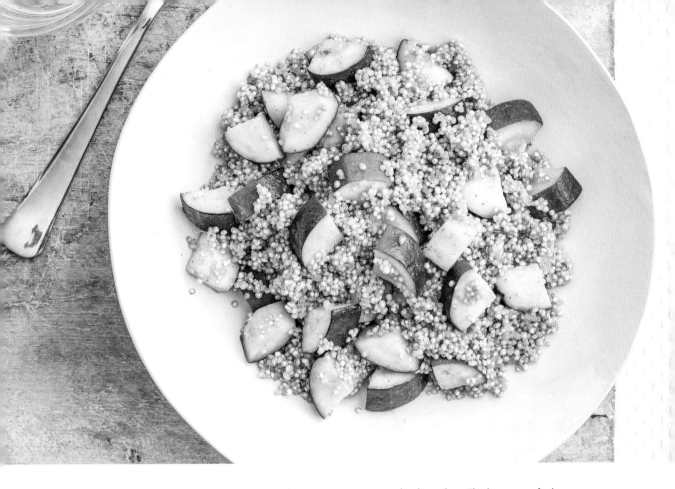

will heal your emotional and physical body with these methods. Consistency and devotion will become your new best friends. The more consistent you are with your lifestyle and habits, the more deeply you will heal and the more profound the transformations will become. The more devoted you are to yourself, the more compassion, understanding, and love you will give to yourself and others. This does not mean you have to give up on all the things you currently love, but it does mean you must make room for new ways of thinking and living.

As you work your way through this book, you will pick up new tools to apply to your life. There is no need to change it all at once, focus on one tool a week and make it a habit. Stick to it and slowly but surely you will see your old habits fall away and new ones take their place. The better you feel, the more you'll want to dive into this work. Have compassion for yourself during this process. Be gentle, live slowly.

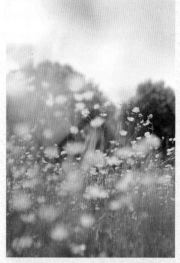

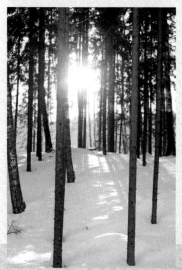

We are all a part of nature. We are of the earth that holds steady beneath us, the fire that brings warmth from above, the flowing water that fills our oceans, the air that breathes life into our lungs, and the ether that pours into the spaces of the unseen.

chapter 1

CONSTITUTION: THE ENERGETICS OF YOUR UNIQUE BEING AND THE THREE DOSHAS

Are you ready to dive deeply into who you are? This chapter will help you begin to understand what makes you special–what makes you innately you–starting by keeping a wellness journal. You will then begin to understand the energetics that make up your unique being. From this point forward, the functions of your body, mind, and spirit will begin to show clarity.

Your Wellness Journal

To know how to treat yourself, you first need to be aware of what you are trying to achieve. Understanding the things that will bring you into and out of balance is the key here. Taking a step back and looking at your life as one big picture is a great exercise to help you see where you need to improve and where you are doing great.

Keeping a journal for at least a three-day period is something I recommend to all my clients at the beginning of their wellness journeys. This allows us to pick apart each category of their health and happiness, generally starting with food and lifestyle. I also have them log the activities they engage in. This is very important because the environment around us and what we choose to expose ourselves to has a huge impact on our health. For example, if you work in a toxic environment, with negative people and high-pressure energy, this will have an effect on your mind, body, and spirit. Lastly, I ask my clients to record when and how they sleep since sleep is crucial for a balanced body and mind.

All these components play a part in your health. Once you understand your unique constitution, you can begin to acknowledge and notice what brings you out of balance and what makes you feel your best. My goal is to give you the tools you need to make a balanced and healthy lifestyle accessible.

Make three copies of the journal page provided (see opposite), then fill one in per day in as much detail as possible. Once you have filled out three days (you always have the option to continue keeping a journal if you like the activity), review what you have written.

This will give you an inside look at how you truly feel, what's aggravating you, what is working, and where your imbalance may be. The more honest and specific you are, the more beneficial this practice will be to your healing journey. You can come back to this journaling practice whenever you'd like to review the progress you've made with the tools from this book.

Here are the types of things you should include in your journal notes:

- **Sleep:** Make a note of any dreams you have, how many times you wake up, the quality of your sleep, and how you feel when you wake up.
- **Food and meal schedules:** Include what you have eaten and when, how you feel emotionally and physically after you have eaten.
- **Daily activities:** Log activities such as sports, working out, going out, drinking, smoking, and dancing and add notes about how they make you feel.
- **Exercise:** Be specific and note what emotional and physical responses are triggered when you exercise.
- **Bowel movements** (this is for your eyes only!): Record how you feel. Make a note of what your stool looks like (stiff, fully formed, mucus in it, or loose, for example). Document this every time you go to the toilet throughout the day.
- **Thoughts and memorable emotions:** Write down anything that stands out to you, anything that made you feel out of balance or really good. Be time specific!

DAY NUMBER:

Sleep:

_____
_____
_____
_____
_____
_____
_____
_____
_____
_____

Food and meal schedules:

_____
_____
_____
_____
_____
_____
_____
_____

Daily activities:

_____
_____
_____
_____
_____
_____
_____
_____

Exercise:

_____
_____
_____
_____
_____
_____
_____
_____
_____

Bowel movements:

_____
_____
_____
_____
_____
_____
_____
_____

Thoughts and
memorable emotions:

_____
_____
_____
_____
_____
_____
_____
_____

Understanding Energetics: Applying Energy to Everyday Living

Energy is in us and all around us. Energy affects all living things, from you to your cat, the bugs in the grass and the grass itself, right down to the tiniest microscopic atom. Ayurveda believes that each living thing contains a balance of five elements: Earth, Air, Fire, Water, and Ether (space). These elements play important roles in balancing our physical and nonphysical bodies. They are energetic forces that affect all the things we do on a daily basis, including the food we eat, our thought patterns, our environment, the type of sleep we have, the way we move our bodies, our digestion, and so on. Think of these energetic elements as a metaphor for the processes that occur within your body. Once you start to understand and feel the interactions of these subtle energies in your body, and in your life, you can begin to balance yourself.

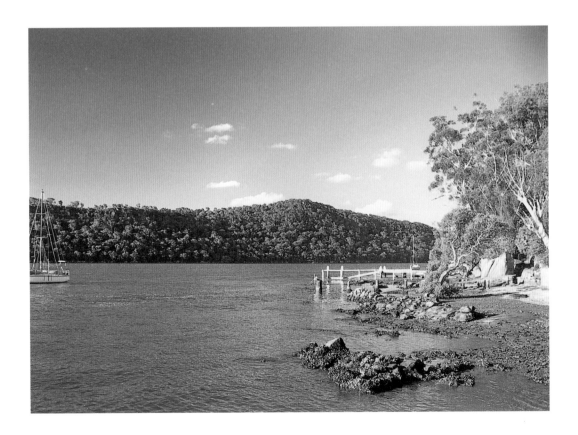

The Three Doshas

In order to experience balance, first we must get to the root of our nature and what makes us unique in the world. Ayurveda believes that the five energetic elements make up the three doshas: Vata, Pitta, and Kapha. Not only are these doshas present in our bodies but also they can be found in the changing seasons, the food we eat, the activities we do, the relationships we have, and the environment we live in.

The three doshas can be used to define the energetic balance of our being. The unique doshic balance inside each of us is determined at the point of conception and stays the same throughout our lives. However, it can be thrown off by internal and external factors, which is why we need to work on balancing our bodies and minds through practices that are right for our individual mind-body type. Our doshic balance affects our likes and dislikes, our emotional and mental tendencies, our physical characteristics, our tendencies toward specific habits, and how vulnerable we are to disease. Once you start to recognize that the energetic elements within your body–and in nature– are composed of the three doshas, you have begun to understand the concept of Ayurveda.

   The charts on the following pages show the natural characteristics, states, and tendencies of each of the doshas. Please refer back to these charts for clarification at any time along your journey.

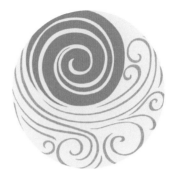

VATA

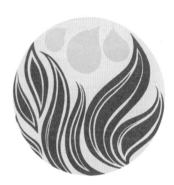

PITTA

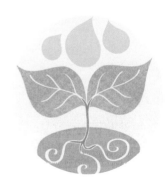

KAPHA

VATA

Governs: All bodily movement.

Elements: Air and Ether (space).

Elemental qualities: Cold, dry, light, swift, mobile, irregular, and rough.

Seasons: Late fall (autumn) and early winter.

Body parts: Small intestine, large intestine, and colon.

Physical features: Individuals with a Vata nature have a predominance of the Air element. This makes Vatas thin, with a light and wiry structure, long angular features, and small dark eyes that are usually brown. Vatas tend to have a small mouth, thin lips, irregular teeth, and receding gums. They may have irregularity in bones, teeth, hair, and spine. They have thin, coarse hair, which is often kinky. Their skin is usually dark and dry. They may have rough skin and lips and/or dry eyes.

Sensitivities: Extreme sensitivity to cold, wind, and dry weather. Cold extremities, such as hands, feet, and nose.

PITTA

Governs: The transformation of food and ideas.

Elements: Fire and Water.

Elemental qualities: Hot, oily, light, liquid, mobile, sharp/precise, soft, and smooth.

Seasons: Summer.

Body parts: Liver, spleen, gallbladder, stomach, duodenum, and pancreas.

Physical features: Individuals with a Pitta nature have a predominance of the Fire element. This makes Pittas hot in constitution with a robust circulation that leads to ruddy coloring and warm extremities. Pittas tend to have a medium-sized build and moderate muscle tone. Their skin is usually fair, warm, reddish, soft, and moist. They have many freckles and moles and a tendency toward rashes and acne. Their eyes are medium-sized and light in color. They have soft, thin, light-colored or reddish hair that may turn gray or bald early.

Sensitivities: Sensitive to heat and humidity. Burn easily in the sun.

KAPHA

Governs: The structure of the body and the formation of all seven tissues: nutritive fluid, blood, muscle, fat, bones, marrow, and reproductive tissues.

Elements: Water and Earth.

Elemental qualities: Cool, wet, oily, heavy, stable, dense, and static.

Seasons: Late winter and early spring.

Body parts: Sinuses, nostrils, throat, bronchi, and lungs.

Physical features: Individuals of a Kapha nature have a predominance of the Water element, which is reflected in their full, soft features and thick, cool, moist skin. Kaphas tend to have a stocky build, a large frame, well-lubricated joints, a well-developed chest, and a strong and well-proportioned body. Kaphas have a tendency to be overweight and they have trouble losing weight. They have thick, soft, oily hair that is often wavy and plentiful. Their eyes are usually large and attractive, blue or light brown in color, with long thick lashes. They tend to have large, round faces with full lips and big white teeth.

Body functions: Erratic appetite and irregular digestion that is easily disturbed. Irregular menstrual cycles. May experience dryness in the form of constipation. Acute premenstrual pain and emotional mood swings. Body aches and stomach aches. Sudden weight loss.

Sleep cycles: Light, restless sleep. May suffer from insomnia.

Personality and mental activities: Vatas have very active and restless mind. They are creative and artistic people whose imaginative ideas can alter direction as frequently as the wind changes direction. They are open and tolerant of others. Adaptable and quick to act, they usually make decisions easily but may struggle with bigger decisions. Vatas have sensitive natures and can retreat when anxious or emotionally insecure. Hyperactive and energetic, Vatas often have multiple ongoing projects. They may have trouble finishing projects because their energy often jumps all over the place and is never fixed or focused on one thing, which can lead them to be unable to complete goals. They may suffer from mental anxiety, worry, and confusion.

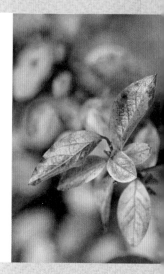

Body functions: Prone to inflammation of muscle tissues, especially in the shoulders and middle of the back where stress accumulates. Robust, healthy appetite. Pittas will become irritable if they skip a meal. Best digestion of all three doshas when balanced. Regular menstrual cycles with heavy bleeding and PMS. May experience profuse sweating, hot flashes, bad breath, and strong body odor. Often suffer from acid build-up and indigestion/heartburn.

Sleep cycles: Light but moderately good sleep. Often overheat during sleep. They burn the candle at both ends, so may suffer from exhaustion and are more likely to experience adrenal fatigue in the long run.

Personality and mental activities: Pittas are intelligent, powerful, and clear, with a focused mind that makes it easy for them to succeed. They are aggressive and competitive in nature. They are workaholics, overly ambitious, and may have a quick temper. With a high energy level, Pittas are sharp and quick-witted, with dynamic personalities. They are great conversationalists. Pittas are content with the direction of their life. They are compassionate and fair.

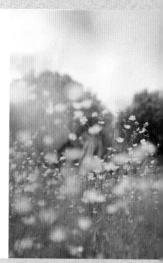

Sensitivities: Intolerant of cold and damp environments.

Body functions: Tendency toward colds, congestion, allergies, and respiratory illnesses. Steady appetite, although may overeat, with slow but regular bowel movements and minimal urination. Water retention, weight gain, and depression are often a complaint. Regular menstrual cycles with little pain and a minimum of premenstrual depression.

Sleep cycles: Kapha types are heavy sleepers; sometimes they like to oversleep, causing sluggishness.

Personality and mental activities: Kaphas are easygoing, fun loving, grounded, and patient. They speak and move slowly. Their calm, reliable nature makes them ideal managers and caretakers. Kaphas have the most energy of all the doshas. With a nonjudgmental nature, they are affectionate and forgiving. They have a stable mind and emotions, and strong endurance. They may sometimes become overly sentimental and may find change difficult. They make attachments easily but can be possessive. They sometimes withdraw from social situations.

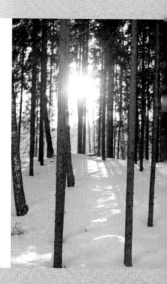

Your Unique Energetic Makeup

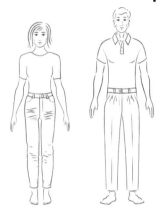

Vata body types

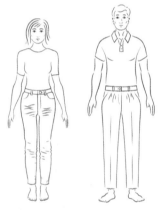

Pitta body types

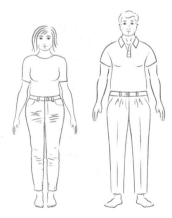

Kapha body types

Now that you have a simple understanding of each dosha, you are ready to find out your own doshic mind-body type.

Ayurveda is unique because it works with each person's body, treating and addressing every individual combination of the three doshas. Since each person has an individual balance of Vata, Pitta, and Kapha, it is important to understand and focus on your own balance (or body type). Take the following quiz to learn which doshic quality you have most of. For the most accurate results, focus on your life as a whole and not your present imbalances or new habits. For each attribute, check the answer that best fits your long-term experience. Once you have completed the quiz, add up the check marks in each of the columns and put the totals in the boxes at the end of the quiz. This will reveal your mind-body type.

Generally, each person has one or two dominant doshas, in rare cases some people are considered tri-doshic, which means they have an equal balance of all three doshas. If you think that this is the case for you, try to apply the tools you learn about all three doshas to the areas of your life that need balancing. For example, if you are in a climate where the seasons change you will have to work year-round to shift your habits to balance all three doshas, since they are equally sensitive in your body. Opposite energies balance each other. If you are hot you will need to balance with cold, if you are damp you will need to balance with dry, and so on.

Once you've discovered your unique constitution, you can begin to alter your lifestyle and diet to optimize your energy levels and maintain a life of balance.

Physical attributes	Vata		Pitta		Kapha	
Body size	Slim	☑	Medium	☐	Large	☐
Body weight	Low	☑	Medium	☐	Overweight	☐
Chin	Angular	☑	Tapering	☐	Rounded	☐
Cheeks	Concave	☐	Flat	☑	Plump	☐
Eyes	Dry, active	☐	Bright, sensitive to light	☐	Big, calm	☑
Lips	Dry, cracked	☑	Red	☐	Smooth, pale	☐
Skin	Thin, dry	☐	Smooth, oily, warm	☑	Thick	☐
Neck	Long, thin	☑	Medium	☐	Short, thick	☐
Chest	Narrow	☑	Medium	☐	Expanded	☐
Stomach	Flat	☑	Medium	☐	Full	☐
Hips	Slender	☐	Medium	☐	Wide	☑
Joints	Crack often, dry	☐	Medium	☑	Large	☐
Appetite	Irregular	☐	Strong	☑	Slow but steady	☐
Digestion	Irregular	☐	Quick	☑	Prolonged	☐
Preferred tastes (see pages 36–37)	Sweet, sour, salty	☑	Sweet, bitter, astringent	☐	Bitter, pungent, astringent	☐
Thirst	Changeable	☑	Surplus	☐	Sparse	☐
Elimination	Constipation	☐	Quick	☑	Sparse, incomplete	☐

Mental and emotional attributes	Vata		Pitta		Kapha	
Mental activity	Very active	☐	Moderate	☐	Slow, methodical	☑
Emotions	Anxiety, fear, uncertainty	☑	Anger, hate, jealousy	☐	Calm, greed, attachment	☑
Intellect	Quick	☐	Precise	☑	Slow, exact	☐
Recollection	Recent good, remote poor	☐	Distinct	☑	Slow and sustained	☐
Mental activity	Quick mind, restless	☐	Sharp intellect, aggressive	☐	Calm, steady, stable	☑
Thoughts	Constantly changing	☐	Fairly steady	☑	Steady, stable, fixed	☐
Concentration	Short-term focus is best	☐	Better-than-average mental concentration	☑	Good ability for long-term focus	☐
Ability to learn	Quick grasp of learning	☑	Medium to moderate grasp of learning	☑	Slow to learn new things	☐
Dreams	Fearful, flying, running, jumping	☐	Angry, fiery, violent, adventurous	☐	Water, clouds, relationships, romance	☑
Sleep	Interrupted, light	☐	Sound, medium	☐	Sound, heavy, long	☑
Speech	Fast, sometimes missing words	☐	Fast, sharp, clear-cut	☐	Slow, clear, sweet	☑
Voice	High pitched	☐	Medium pitched	☑	Low pitched	☐

Important

If you are unsure of your dosha after taking the quiz, start to carry out some of the practices in this book and come back to the quiz after you've begun making positive changes in your lifestyle.

Behavioral profile	Vata		Pitta		Kapha	
Eating speed	Quick	☐	Medium	☐	Slow	☑
Hunger level	Irregular	☐	Sharp, needs food when hungry	☑	Can easily miss meals	☐
Food and drink	Prefer warm food and drink	☑	Prefer cold food and drink	☐	Prefer dry and warm food and drink	☐
Achieving goals	Easily distracted	☐	Focused and driven	☐	Slow and steady	☑
Giving donations	Give small amounts	☐	Give nothing or very infrequently	☑	Give regularly and generously	☐
Relationships	Many casual relationships	☐	Intense relationships	☐	Long and deep relationships	☑
Sex drive	Variable or low	☐	Moderate	☑	Strong	☐
Works best	While supervised	☐	Alone	☑	In groups	☐
Weather preferences	Strongly dislike the cold	☑	Strongly dislike the heat	☐	Strongly dislike cool and wet	☐
Reaction to stress	Get excited quickly	☑	Get excited moderately	☐	Get excited slowly	☐
Financial	Don't save, spend quickly	☐	Save, but big spender	☑	Save regularly, accumulate wealth	☐
Friendships	Tend toward short-term friendships, make friends quickly	☐	Tend toward medium-term friendships	☐	Tend to form long-lasting friendships	☑

Totals

	Vata	Pitta	Kapha
	13	*17*	*12*

Once you have completed the quiz, add up the check marks in each of the columns and put the total in the boxes at the end of the quiz. The column with the most check marks indicates your primary dosha.

Lifestyle and Food Recommendations for the Doshas

If you take away two things from this book let it be your unique constitution and these simple recommendations on how to keep your balance through food and lifestyle practices. The advice below is easy to incorporate into your lifestyle, regardless of your doshic imbalance/balance. Try and incorporate some of it as you move along on your wellness journey.

 RECOMMENDATIONS FOR VATA

- Cultivate calmness and stability in your life by establishing routines.
- Take time away from your busy lifestyle and increase your body-mind connection by meditating daily, getting regular massages, particularly Thai yoga massages, grounding yourself by walking on the earth barefoot, or attending restorative yoga and Pilates classes.
- Reduce excess stimulation, including noise, distractions, and overactivity.
- The best approach to work is to embrace your creativity and communication skills and seek work that is less competitive and physically demanding because Vatas are most sensitive to highly stressful situations and environments.
- Eat frequent routine meals, particularly nourishing, well-cooked food served warm.
- Sweet, sour, and salty tastes are best (see Food Related to Ayurveda: Eating for Your Dosha and Agni, pages 36–40).

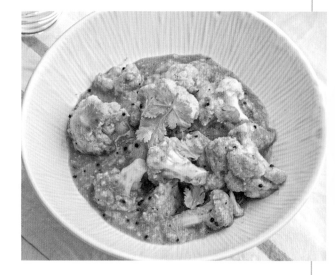

- Eat hearty soups, raw organic dairy products, protein, and grains.
- Avoid foods that are dry, reduce caffeine, and stay away from carbonated drinks.

RECOMMENDATIONS FOR PITTA

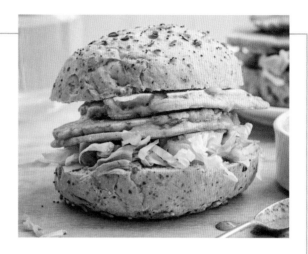

- Moderate exercise and activities such as walking at night or in cooler weather, swimming, jogging, and reading are great for Pitta.
- Move away from highly competitive activities and those that cause heavy exertion and perspiration.
- Moderate routine in diet, activities, and sleep will help keep Pittas calm and cool.
- Promote a loving and forgiving lifestyle that tries to reduce conflict, aggression, and overcompetitiveness.
- Make time and space to relax outside of work.
- Both cool and warm foods work well for people with a Pitta constitution because of their strong digestive fire. Stay away from foods with too much heat and spice.
- Sweet, bitter, and astringent tastes are best.

- Fill your diet with fruits, vegetables, beans, and grains.
- Avoid foods that are spicy, salty, fermented, and sour. Avoid vinegar, ketchup, coffee and other forms of caffeine, and too much meat and alcohol.

RECOMMENDATIONS FOR KAPHA

- Stimulating exercise and activities that work up a good sweat without leaving you exhausted are great. Try Pilates, vigorous yoga, high-intensity interval training (HIIT), running, endurance sports, etc. Change up your routine to keep the energy vibrant.
- Promote a lifestyle that wakens the mind and breaks up inactivity while creating a loving space and compassionate support that regulates and reduces attachments.
- Strong interpersonal skills and compassion help Kaphas to be good providers and managers.
- It's advisable to incorporate physical exertion and discipline in your job.
- Reduce the amount of food you eat at each meal. As a rule of thumb, try to only eat as much food as would fit in the palm of your hand.
- Pungent, bitter, and astringent tastes are best.

- Choose warm, light, and dry foods. The liberal use of hot spices is recommended. Vegetables, beans, and dry grains are also recommended.
- Whole grains, oils, and nuts are not recommended. Avoid dairy, meat, and sweet foods.

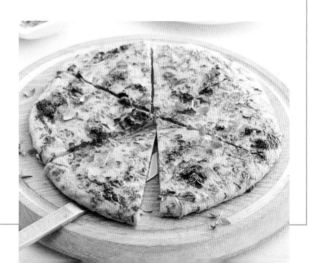

Eating a diet specific to your unique constitution will make you feel alive and abundant. Processed foods are made with dead energy. Living foods, picked from Mother Earth, grow for us so we become one with nature.

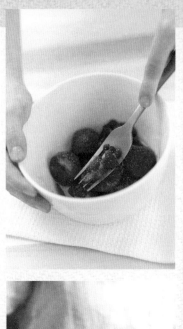

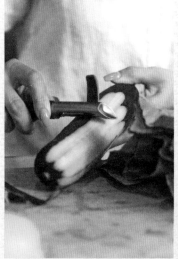

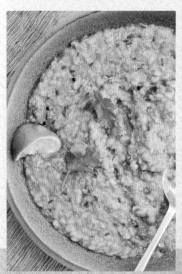

chapter 2

NUTRITION: FOOD BRINGS BALANCE TO OUR BODIES

Ayurveda views nutrition as an integral part of the self-healing process. This aspect of daily living is one that we have complete control over. In this chapter, you will learn that dieting does not work and living with an awareness around food is what brings balance to our bodies.

Food as Medicine

Are you ready to shift your perspective on food? Food is our most available medicine. What if instead of looking to the latest fad diet or supplement to change your body, skin, or hair, for example, you look to the food you eat to make those changes?

I wholeheartedly promote the use of herbs and superfoods to boost health and wellness, but nutrition needs to come first. The next time you sit down for a meal, order food at a restaurant, or cook at home, I urge you to ask yourself the following question: "What is this food giving me?" If you're not sure of the answer, you should consider that as a clear sign that you could make a change in your life without spending lots of money on supplements and relying on them to do the job food could be doing for you. If you want to see a change, you have to make a change!

When you go beyond looking at food as flavor in your mouth and start to view it as fuel, you begin to see what your body needs. Based on your dosha and the information you've learned so far, do you think you are eating foods that are balancing to your body type?

The number one piece of advice I give to all of my clients is to keep it simple. Even if you don't have access to food that is fit for your constitution 100 percent of the time, keep it simple. When it comes to the food you are eating, keep the ingredients to a minimum, less is often more. If you put too many ingredients and complicated sauces and spices on your plate they can cause symptoms such as bloating, gas, indigestion, candida, and ulcers. The closer you are to eating food in its natural form, the better you will feel.

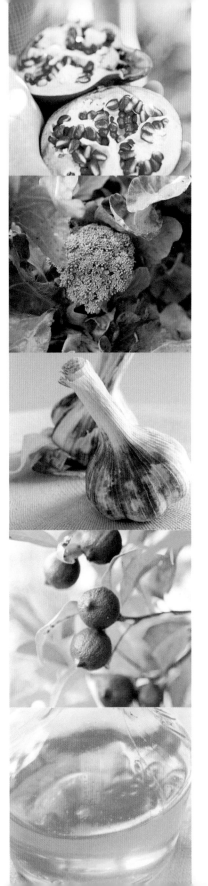

Healthy Food Swaps

Another way to transition into healthier eating habits is to make simple food swaps. It's important to select food that is as close as possible to its natural form because some products that are advertised as being "healthy" are completely modified, filled with hidden sugars, stabilizers, gums, and unnecessary additives. Eating unhealthy foods that are marketed as "healthy" won't make you sick or unhealthy the first time you eat them, but if you consume them on a regular basis they will start to damage your body.

We either eat our food as medicine or we eat our medicine as food. It's wise to ask yourself the following questions when buying new products or grocery shopping:

- Where does this food come from?
- What is this food made out of?
- Will this food serve me on my healing journey?
- Is this food right for my body type?

Watch out for the following marketing angles when buying food:

- Gluten free
- Cholesterol free
- Fat free
- Whole grain
- Sugar free
- Organic
- All natural

Just because a product is described with some of those words does not mean the food is healthy or pure. Organic candy is still candy. Yes, whole-grain food is great, but what else is in there? Always read the labels.

You are your best weapon when it comes to combating illness and keeping your body healthy. Use your knowledge to your advantage: scrutinize labels, research the ingredients if you don't know what they are, and make the best choices you possibly can. Next are some examples of healthy food swaps.

Fiber Snacks

Fiber bars aren't real food. They are designed for convenience, yes, but what is convenient about not getting nutrients from your food? Fiber bars are high in added sugars and low in nutrients. Remember, our mission is to eat to fuel our bodies, and this is not going to happen if we feed them with imitation foods that have empty calories and no or low nutrients.

A great swap for fiber bars is fruit; berries to be precise. Berries are the real place you'll find bioavailable fiber. They are packed with

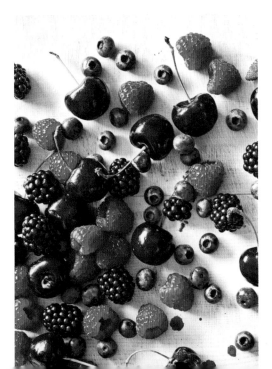

antioxidants, vitamins, minerals, water, and natural fiber and they are low in sugar and calories. Berries make a wonderful snack for Kapha and Pitta types. If you're looking for high-fiber foods, you'll find that the highest form of fiber is going to come from food in its natural form rather than food that has been processed and turned into something else. Nutrient-dense and fiber-rich foods such as raspberries, strawberries, avocados, nuts, and oats can all be found in nature.

Cooking Oils

It's understandable that most people believe that vegetable and canola (rapeseed) oils are safe to consume because we are constantly fed misinformation about the foods we consume, which leaves many people in the dark. These oils are highly processed, refined, heated, bleached, and deodorized. The amount of high heat these oils are subjected to during industrial processing (just to be bottled) has a negative impact on the healthy compounds in the oils and the finished products are ultimately stripped of their omega-3 fatty acids.

Canola oil can be found in many prepared foods, even in the health-food stores. It can even be found in some forms of dried fruit! Always read the food labels and try to opt for a heathier form of oil. Extra virgin olive oil is a good swap. It is produced by cold-pressing (a process that avoids high-heat treatments), which leaves it full of heart-healthy fats.

Canola and vegetable oils can be found in fake butter substitutes as well. Instead of buying those, opt for a healthier and more nourishing option such as ghee. Ghee has a high smoking point, is packed with omega fatty acids, and is full of vitamins A, D, E, and K. For those who are lactose intolerant, ghee is great because the milk fat is cooked out of it,

leaving it lactose free! Always buy organic oils. Rancid or overly processed oils can aggravate Pitta.

Sweeteners

Agave sweetener has been advertised as healthy but unfortunately it doesn't really live up to the standards that the food industry is holding it to. Although agave sweetener is better than white sugar and other processed forms of sugarcane, it is highly refined and the end product contains large amounts of fructose, which is an inflammatory and damaging form of sugar. A healthy swap for agave sweetener is organic maple syrup. Maple syrup is much less processed, it is high in antioxidants and magnesium, and it tastes amazing.

If you don't like maple syrup, you could also swap raw honey for agave sweetener. When buying honey, it's crucial to select raw honey, which is rich in gut-healing enzymes, high in antioxidants, and barely processed. Heating raw honey changes its medicinal properties, so never add raw honey to hot liquids—wait until they have cooled to a warm temperature.

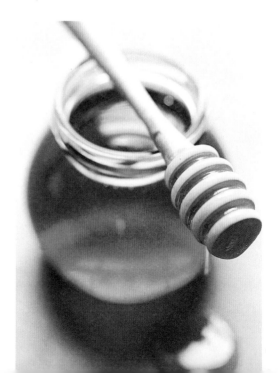

Other possible swaps are monk fruit sugar and stevia. Choose stevia in its raw form or a minimally processed form like the one recommended on page 157. Stevia is much sweeter than agave sweetener and processed sugar, so only use a little at a time.

Flour

Wheat flour is often advertised as being "enriched," which essentially means the product was stripped of its natural nutrients and then those nutrients were added back to the flour in a synthetic way. Once this has happened, the flour is toxic. White flour is highly processed, refined, and bleached by applying chlorine dioxide. Not only is it low in fiber but also it will inevitably lead to unnecessary and unhealthy weight gain, congestion, inflammation, and bloating. The unfortunate truth is that even the "healthiest" food products often contain seemingly harmless white flour.

Almond flour is much less processed than white flour and can be swapped in almost all recipes with minor or no adjustments to the rest of the recipe. Almond flour is higher in fiber, protein, and healthy fats than white flour. It is great for those Kapha types who need an easily digestible carbohydrate. Other swap options are oat, millet, brown rice, coconut, chickpea, and tapioca flours. If you're looking for a swap for white bread, try Ezekiel bread (sprouted grain bread), paleo bread, or sprouted sourdough.

Salad Toppings

You'll find croutons in most Caesar salads. Most people think that croutons are healthy because they are part of a salad. Wrong! They are actually made from white bread, cooked in highly processed oils, contain little to no protein, and have less fiber than nuts. This is why a healthy, crunchy swap for salad croutons is raw sprouted nuts, such as almonds, pistachios, walnuts, and macadamia nuts. They contain no damaged fats, are full of antioxidants, and are high in fiber, good fats, and protein, plus they will keep you satisfied for longer.

Cheese

Processed cheese is full of added hormones, genetically modified ingredients, and chemicals, and it doesn't even resemble real cheese. Even blocks of real cheese are not that great unless they are unpasteurized and raw. This is because pasteurization kills the natural good bacteria and enzymes that help us breakdown the proteins and fats in dairy products. Too much dairy can cause inflammation and mucus build-up in the body, especially if you don't have a microbiome (healthy gut bacteria that breaks down food and protects against germs) that is strong enough to digest it.

Raw-milk cheese is a wonderful swap for processed cheese. However, most of us don't have access to raw-milk cheese, which is why the real swap goes to nutritional yeast. It tastes great on salads and in soups and it is also a good way to add a cheese-like flavor to sauces. Nutritional

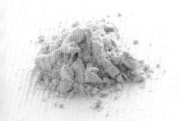
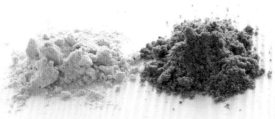
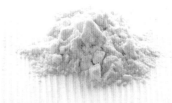

yeast contains 50–100 percent of your daily requirement of B vitamins and it is high in protein and fiber.

If you are predominantly a Kapha type, stay away from dairy altogether and use nutritional yeast instead. Vatas are aggravated by dry-aged cheeses, which can cause constipation, and should replace them with a soft probiotic nut cheese, which is actually much easier to find and make than you think (see Cashew Cream Sauce, page 85).

Flavoring

I know flavored coffee can be yummy but there are many ways to get the flavor you desire from natural food sources instead of flavored coffee creamers. Coffee creamers often contain unhealthy oils, thickeners, preservatives, sweeteners, and dangerous emulsifiers that degrade our precious gut mucosa. Drinking a substance like this can cause many different digestive upsets, one of which is leaky gut syndrome.

Healthy swaps for coffee creamer are coconut cream, ghee, and coconut oil, believe it or not. All three alternatives contain the healthiest form of fat available with no added sugar or emulsifiers. The best way to make flavored coffee is to blend about ½ teaspoon of your chosen alternative creamer in your coffee.

If you would like to add extra flavor to your coffee, like French vanilla, hazelnut, or toffee, I suggest buying flavored stevia drops (see Resources, page 157, for my suggested brands) or using spices such as cinnamon, cardamom, nutmeg, or even raw cacao. All these options are natural and safe to use.

Store-bought Jam

I know jam can be convenient and cheap but jam is not fruit, jam is not healthy. Commercially produced store-bought jam not only contains loads of added sugar but also contains ingredients like high-fructose corn syrup and other preservatives. There are maybe a handful of jam brands that use real fruit, apple juice to sweeten, and citric acid to preserve. These "more natural" options are still not ideal, though. I would recommend them over the others if you have to buy jam in a store–but you don't.

To be honest, unless you're getting your jam straight from a farm, I suggest swapping out jam altogether and replacing it with mashed-up berries. This is a great alternative to jam and it only contains one ingredient. You could even add chia seeds to the berries if you want to get fancy. The chia seeds work a bit like gelatin, absorbing the liquid from the mashed berries to give them a more jam-like quality. Chia seeds are also high in omega fatty acids.

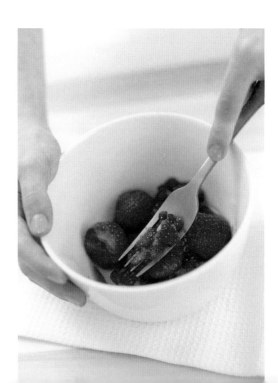

Resolving Your Relationship with Food: Learning How to Eat Intuitively

The beautiful thing about Ayurveda is that it truly teaches you about individualized medicine. It instructs you not to compare yourself to others and recommends that you follow the natural rhythms already inside your being and–above all–become more intuitive in your daily life. I hope by now you are beginning to understand that you are in control of this journey: you make the decisions, you take the lead when it comes to your own body.

Intuitive eating is about having freedom around food. You can eat what you want, when you want without guilt, shame, sickness, bingeing, or triggering negative thought patterns. Practice intuitive eating by paying attention to how food makes you feel, how much food you want and need to eat, what food you actually enjoy, and what food affects your moods and physical body. This is intuitive eating with Ayurveda. The more you become acquainted with your body, the better you will feel. Your body wants to trust that you will fill it with balanced fuel; it actually gives you the ability to make the right decisions. Over time, it's common for our bodies to lose trust in our ability to nourish them. Letting go of the fear of who you truly are beneath the diets, labels, body image, and more will help you become happier and healthier in body, mind, and spirit.

Diet vs Intuitive Eating

The first myth I'd like to bust about intuitive eating is that it makes you fat and gives you mood swings. This is far from the truth. In fact, you are more likely to gain weight and have mood swings when you deprive your body of what it wants. When you give yourself permission to eat what your body wants and there are no "good" or "bad" foods, it acts like reverse psychology. Now that you can have whatever you want, you don't really want it. Suddenly you can have one bite of something and be done with it, knowing that food is there for you if you want more.

Even though you understand that it's best to follow a lifestyle and nutritional plan that is going to balance your specific body, it's vital to know that you can still indulge in the food and drink you love the most. This is an important factor when it comes to my teachings of Ayurveda. It may not be the most traditional way to approach eating and Ayurveda, but I think it makes sense because we live in a time when we are all really disconnected from our senses, our emotions, and our knowledge of what we truly need. Most of us have grown up in a society that is so attached to image–what we should be and what we should eat–that we have to break the diet mentality to help us get to a place of knowing our own bodies on a deeper level.

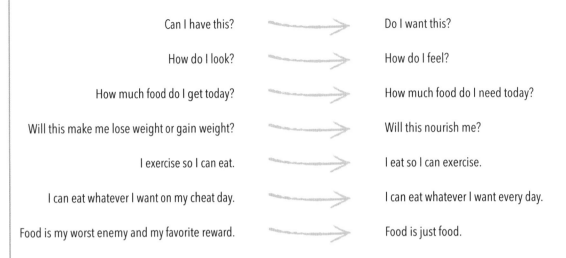

HERE ARE SOME WAYS TO REFOCUS COMMON DIETING ATTITUDES ABOUT FOOD:

Can I have this?	Do I want this?
How do I look?	How do I feel?
How much food do I get today?	How much food do I need today?
Will this make me lose weight or gain weight?	Will this nourish me?
I exercise so I can eat.	I eat so I can exercise.
I can eat whatever I want on my cheat day.	I can eat whatever I want every day.
Food is my worst enemy and my favorite reward.	Food is just food.

Learning to differentiate an emotional or memory craving from a physical craving will help you eat intuitively. When the body needs a nutrient it sends signals to the brain so we eat those nutrients. It's kind of like a car, a little light comes on when it needs to be fueled or needs oil. Unfortunately, we don't have it that easy and we must tune into our bodies and question those signals to understand what we need. If you ever notice yourself craving sugar, instead of letting that craving take over, ask yourself the following questions: What did I eat today? Am I getting enough variety? Is my blood sugar low? Your answers will help you discern what your body is truly signaling you to eat.

There are such thing as beneficial cravings and nonbeneficial cravings. Nonbeneficial cravings are usually linked to our emotional state. They can come up if we aren't nurturing our bodies and can cause feelings of tension, guilt, shame, or regret. If you eat a lot of junk food or skip meals often you may find yourself constantly craving oily, sugary, and processed foods. This can be an indication that you are stuck in a cycle of not feeding your body with nutrient-dense foods. Beneficial cravings mean that you are in control of what you are putting in your body and your emotions are not driving you to eat.

Our intuition is a great guide when it comes to making the best choices for ourselves. To implement this, start to notice what's going on in your body and mind when you crave a specific food. The more conscious and aware you are, the more you can nurture your body. When we trust our internal body cues over external diet rules we can begin to move and flow through life with more ease.

The beauty of integrating Ayurveda with intuitive eating methods is that you become a powerhouse of knowledge and can start living from a place of full enjoyment. Each dosha has its own eating guidelines to help heal and balance the body but this doesn't mean you are never again allowed to eat other foods. Once you know your dosha and understand how your body's energy naturally ebbs and flows, intuitively you will know which of the energetic elements within your body are out of balance and be equipped with the tools to help bring yourself back into balance.

Focus on learning the energetic qualities of all types of food, rather than simply studying a list of ingredients suitable for Vata, Pitta, or Kapha as if you are memorizing a diet plan. You need to know what all food can do, not just the food that you might need because of your main dosha. If you eat with a purpose, there is no need to restrict or diet. When you do impose restrictions or cut out entire food groups, your body can go into shock, which can cause more imbalances (another reason that diets don't work). The information about food that comes from Ayurveda will provide you with tools that can be applied to anyone's life. Remember, these are tools not rules.

Indulging in your favorite food is okay. It's inevitable that you will indulge from time to time because this is a lifestyle not a temporary diet. This is a long-term process. There will be times when you decide you want to eat a piece of cake made with sugar, flour, and butter even though your constitution will not agree with eating that cake. You need to throw out everything you've ever been taught about diets and restrictions. You need to address your relationship with food and learn your body's signals. If you are feeling out of balance and have been overindulging, this is not an excuse to indulge further. Be honest and real with yourself about your habits and your health. Don't allow yourself to feel sick because emotionally you are out of balance and placating those feelings with food. That is not intuitive eating, that is emotional eating; they are two different things.

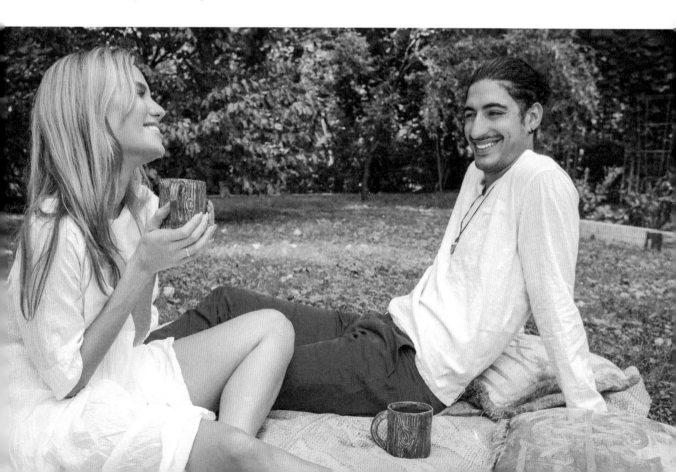

Food Related to Ayurveda

In Ayurveda, food is categorized by its energetic qualities, how it affects each dosha, and its taste. *Rasa* is the Sanskrit word for "taste." Opposite you will find a chart that breaks down food into six different rasas: sweet, sour, salty, pungent, bitter, and astringent. These tastes are important because each one can cause either balance or imbalance to a dosha.

The principal of "like attracts like" can be helpful when trying to understand the concept of the six tastes. For example, Pitta types generally love spicy or pungent foods, but if they eat too much of either they will become out of balance and may suffer from indigestion, heartburn, and skin rashes. Likewise, if Vata types eat too many drying, cold, and raw foods they will become out of balance and most likely experience bloating and gas. And if Kapha types eat too many creamy, heavy, and sweet foods, over time they will form an imbalance that could lead to weight gain, lethargy, and excess mucus build-up. Imbalances are often an initial cause of the food we eat.

Eating For Your Dosha

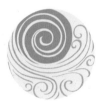

TIPS FOR VATA

- Sweet, salty, and sour tastes, as well as warm, oily, and heavy food, are best for Vata.
- Increase warm, nourishing, and grounding food.
- Try soups with ginger and fennel as a snack or lunch.
- Minimize raw, cold, and dry foods.

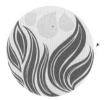

TIPS FOR PITTA

- Sweet, bitter, and astringent tastes are best for Pitta.
- Increase cooling and calming food.
- Try infusing room-temperature drinking water with cilantro (coriander) and cucumber.
- Minimize hot, spicy, and oily food.

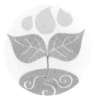

TIPS FOR KAPHA

- Pungent, bitter, and astringent tastes are best for Kapha.
- Increase cleansing and drying food.
- Try a chickpea and kale salad for lunch.
- Minimize heavy foods, salt, dairy, and sweet foods.

Increasing a Dosha

To increase a dosha means to aggravate it. If you aggravate a dosha too many times you can start to build up a long-term imbalance. However, if you are out of balance and your dosha is low, you will need to increase the dosha in order to bring yourself back into balance.

THE SIX TASTES

Taste	Food	Effect on mind-body physiology
Sweet	Whole grains, wheat, rice, cereals, starchy vegetables, dairy, meat, chicken, fish, sugar, honey, molasses, dates, licorice root.	Soothing effect on the body. Brings satisfaction and also builds body mass. Balances Vata and Pitta. Excessive intake can aggravate Kapha.
Sour	Tomatoes, citrus fruit, berries, vinegars, pickled foods, fermented foods, tamarind, wine, salad dressings.	Stimulates the appetite and aids digestion but can be irritating to those suffering from heartburn. Balances Vata. Excessive intake will aggravate Pitta and Kapha.
Salty	Sea vegetables, sea salt, Himalayan salt, rock salt, tamari, soy sauce, black olives, salted meat, fish.	Enhances the appetite and intensifies other tastes. Balances Vata. Too much salt increases Kapha and Pitta.
Pungent	Hot peppers, onions, garlic, ginger, mustard, hot spices, cayenne pepper, black pepper, cloves, salsas.	Promotes sweating and clears lymph and sinus passages. Balances Kapha. Excessive intake aggravates Vata and Pitta.
Bitter	Raw green vegetables, green leafy vegetables, green and yellow vegetables, kale, celery, broccoli, sprouts, beets (beetroot), turmeric, green tea, black tea.	Detoxifies the entire body system. Decreases water retention. Balances Kapha and Pitta. Excessive intake increases Vata and may cause some gas or indigestion.
Astringent	Green beans, alfalfa sprouts, okra, cauliflowers, lentils, dried beans, unripe bananas, green grapes, grape skins, pomegranates, figs, cranberries, green apples, tea.	Dry cleansing action. Decongests. Absorbs excess moisture and may cause excessive dryness in the mouth. Balances Kapha and Pitta. Excessive intake increases Vata.

Agni: Your Digestive Fire

Agni is the Sanskrit word for "fire." When people talk about agni, they are generally referring to the digestive system. Your agni is your digestive fire. Not only does your agni tell you when you are hungry, but it also transforms food into fuel. If your agni doesn't run smoothly, you may experience gas, bloating, indigestion, and ama (a toxic build-up that slows down all bodily systems).

VATA types tend toward a fluctuating agni, one that can be strong at one moment and weak at another. It is very important for Vatas to maintain a steady agni throughout the day so they can avoid fluctuating energy levels.

PITTA types tend to have an intense, fiery agni, one that has the ability to run smoothly when in balance but can quickly be thrown out of balance, creating a hot and acidic agni. Long-term acidic agni can cause heartburn, ulcers, indigestion, and more.

KAPHA types tend to have a slow, wet agni, one that often needs a little help to get going and maintain. The damp and cool nature of Kapha can cause sluggishness and depression if not managed daily.

QUESTIONNAIRE: HOW IS YOUR AGNI DOING?

For each of the following statements, check the box if it applies to your current bodily state. If you check all of the boxes, you know you're in good shape. If not, you know there's room to improve and balance your agni.

My tongue is a healthy pink color, with little to no build-up on top. ☐

My body tells me when I am hungry and I listen. I rarely skip meals. ☐

I poop every morning. ☐

My energy levels don't fluctuate throughout the day and I feel energized without the use of stimulants. ☐

QUESTIONNAIRE: SIGNS AND SYMPTOMS OF AMA

For each of the following statements, check the box if it applies to your current bodily state. If you check all or most of the boxes, you know that your body is out of balance and you have toxins that need to be removed. If none of these apply to you, consider yourself in good condition to focus on other areas.

My tongue is covered with a white or gray coating. ☐

I don't have a consistent meal routine and I can never tell when I'm hungry. ☐

I usually eat when I'm supposed to eat or when I'm feeling emotional rather than when I am hungry. ☐

I almost always overeat. ☐

It is common for me to feel bloated, sluggish, and have pain after eating. ☐

I often fart and/or burp. ☐

I strongly desire to feel more energized. ☐

I often want to eat unhealthy foods and don't know what my body is really craving. ☐

I have a problem with mucus. I am always stuffed up and/or have a lot of phlegm. ☐

How to Keep your Agni and Ama in Balance

Now that you know the state of your agni, here are a few tips to help you keep your agni in balance.

- Eat two to three meals per day according to your dosha. If you experience hunger pains between meals, feel free to snack.

- Eat on a consistent schedule. Try to eat at the same times each day.

- Drink hot water with lemon in between meals and thirty minutes before meals. If you have a Vata or Kapha constitution, try adding both lemon and freshly grated ginger to the water before meals.

- Make lunch the biggest meal of the day, especially if you are having a large amount of protein.

- Have small meals for dinner to avoid exhausting yourself with cooking large meals at the end of the day. If you are still hungry before bed, have a glass of warm almond milk spiced with nutmeg, cinnamon, ginger, and/or cardamom (see, for example, Ashwagandha Chai Latte on page 109).

- Only eat when you are hungry. If you don't feel hungry and find yourself emotionally eating rather than physically eating, notice the sensations that are present for you when hunger is absent. Sometimes you have to train your inner intelligence to wake up and signal your body.

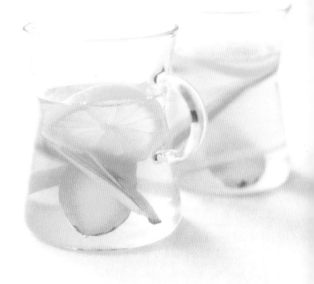

- Agni is highest in the middle of the day (around noon). By the time it is dark, agni is settling down and will be much lower. If you find that you have a weak agni, it's best to follow the natural rhythms of your body and honor where your agni is each day. Don't force yourself to eat when you aren't hungry. It's best to have a warm beverage instead. This way you avoid stressing your digestion and weakening your agni.

Food Combining with Ayurveda

Another way to ensure your agni is working properly, and to avoid digestive disturbances, is to follow Ayurveda's proper food-combining guidelines.

As with everything in Ayurveda, listen to your body, get to know your natural rhythms, and adapt these guidelines to suit your needs. As you embark on this new process of food combining, take note of which food combinations work best for your body type and which are worst. Take the combining slowly so you can really understand, see, and feel what your body needs.

Food combining may seem like a daunting task and can feel overwhelming at times, especially because most cultures don't combine food properly. Poor food combining can lead to an array of digestive issues and a build-up of ama, both things you absolutely don't want.

You will learn more about which food is good to combine in chapter 3, but for now, without making things too complicated, let's go over some common food combinations that are a no-no in Ayurveda.

Tomatoes and Cheese

Tomatoes and cheese are basically a belly bomb of gas and bloat. It's never advisable to combine the two. Food from the nightshade family, including tomatoes, eggplants (aubergines), potatoes, peppers, and goji berries, should rarely be consumed due to the toxic alkaloids they give off during digestion. Alkaloids are basically a defense mechanism some plants have to ward off their predators. Unluckily for us, delicious nightshades have the highest active alkaloids of all plant food. These alkaloids make nightshades very difficult to digest. When paired with cheese, which is already

hard to digest, you have yourself a stressed belly. Nightshades aren't necessarily off limits but it's best to consume them in small portions—and not often because they are disturbing to all three doshas.

Fruit and Milk

Fruit and milk are a pretty common combination, especially if you are into smoothies, milk shakes, or ice-cream. (I definitely had my fair share of strawberries, bananas, and whipped cream as a kid.) Have you ever squeezed a bit of lemon juice into a glass of milk? Probably not, but if you had you would have seen that it curdles and tastes downright awful. The same reaction occurs within our bodies when we combine fruit and milk; things essentially ferment in the stomach. If you are addicted to your fruit smoothies, try opting for coconut milk instead of regular milk.

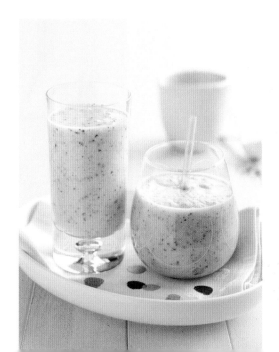

Proteins with Dairy

This is probably the hardest food combination to avoid for most of my clients. It's very common for the two to be served together, particularly when the dairy aspect is cheese, but this combination is actually counterintuitive for the body. Although cheese is known to contain a significant amount of protein, it is not considered a main source of protein in this instance. Meat with cheese, fish with cheese, and even beans with cheese are all poor food combinations and will inevitably lead to digestive disturbances. Protein and cheese are both heavy in nature. Eaten together they are harder to digest than, say, cooked vegetables and cheese in the middle of the afternoon—which, by the way, is a great way (and time) to consume cheese if you like it.

In addition, you shouldn't eat two different types of protein in one meal (an example of this would be beans with fish). This is because the body finds it difficult to digest proteins, so you don't want to slow down digestion even further or create ama by increasing the burden on your digestive system.

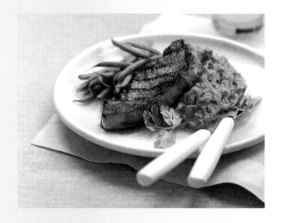

Fruit and Other Food

Fruit should almost always be eaten on its own. There are very few exceptions to this rule, though cooked fruit is one such case. Melon, in particular, should always be eaten on its own and it is best eaten on an empty stomach. (Sorry for bursting your bubble if you love prosciutto and melon; that's another belly bomb!) The easily digestible melon can cause fermentation when it is eaten with other food, which leads to a build-up of bacteria and ama in the stomach if you repeatedly combine melon with other food. If you are currently combining loads of fruit with grains or other foods and have digestive issues, try separating the different types of food and eating them at least twenty minutes apart (fruit first) and see if you feel a change or notice a relief in discomfort.

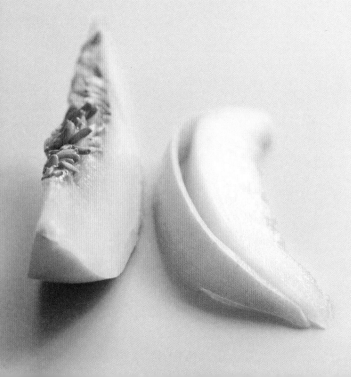

OTHER COMMON COMBINATIONS TO AVOID

Sandwiches: Often combining wheat with meat or raw food (lettuce) with cooked food (meat) and/or fermented food (cheese, sour cream, vinegar), sandwiches can be very difficult to digest.

Cheeseburgers: Wheat, meat, and dairy are difficult enough to digest separately. When combined in a cheeseburger, they confound the stomach.

Yogurt with fruit: Fruit eaten with yogurt will curdle and ferment in the stomach.

Burritos: A lot of ingredients are used to make a burrito. They often combine vegetables with meat, meat with dairy (sour cream and cheese), raw tomatoes with cooked, and generally contain far too many ingredients.

Pizzas: Many pizzas combine wheat with both cheese and tomatoes.

Apples with peanut butter: Peanuts take a long time to digest. While the body churns away at the peanut butter, the bacteria churns away at the fruit. You can swap peanut butter for tahini if you like this combination.

EAT FOOD IN THE RIGHT ORDER

The gut holds onto food until all the nutrition has been extracted so always eat food that is easy to digest first, hard to digest last. For example, eat berries before granola, rice before lentils, steamed veggies before nuts. Every organism loves food that is easy to digest, including the bacteria in our gut. When easy-to-digest food gets stuck behind hard-to-digest food in a traffic jam, the easy-to-digest food ferments.

RULE OF THUMB

- Keep starches and heavy proteins separate.
- Eat fruit on its own or eat fruit at least twenty minutes before other food.
- Keep dairy and proteins separate, and don't combine nightshades (see page 41) with dairy.
- Try not to drink liquids during meals as this will slow down the digestive process and weaken agni. Instead, drink warm water with lemon up to thirty minutes before you eat.

Conscious Eating: Becoming the Ayur-vidya

Eating should be approached as a sacred and sensual experience. You are literally joining energies together. It's important to be mindful and conscious of your eating. *Ayur* means "life or vital power" in Sanskrit, and *Vidya* means "knowledge and clarity"–hence the term Ayur-vidya. Here is a simple yet effective ritual to increase your connection to your food.

1   Before you eat, feel and sense what your body needs and is truly craving. Make decisions about the food you are going to eat based on what is best for your body in that moment and what will serve you long term.

2   Once you have prepared your meal, sit in a calm and quiet environment, draw your attention to the food on your plate, and say a prayer, mantra, or blessing over your food. (I like to remove any negative energy that has been placed upon my food; use my positive radiant light to infuse my meal with strength, gratitude, wisdom, and longevity; and be thankful that I have the means to nourish my being body, mind, and spirit with this food.) One of the main reasons why we say a blessing and infuse our food with positive energy is to help us remember that our food is energy. Food is fuel to nourish our bodies and it's important to honor that.

3   As you eat, slowly breath in through your nose and out through your nose. Deep breathing will help you slow down and feel your food. Not only will you taste your food with heightened senses but also you will gain more energy from it.

4   Use the tools already embedded deep within your body. Chew your food as well as possible. The saliva in your mouth is loaded with digestive enzymes to help you break down your food before you even swallow it.

5   After you've eaten, draw attention to how each part of your body feels:
    * Is the food giving you energy and love?
    * Is your mind being nurtured?
    * Do you feel you are absorbing all the nutrients?
    * Do you feel happy?

Practice this ritual as often as you can. Choosing to be in a calm environment while you eat is choosing to heal your body through the practice of mindful eating. Try to abstain from negative conversation while you are dining with others–this will help your body stay in a calm and neutral state.

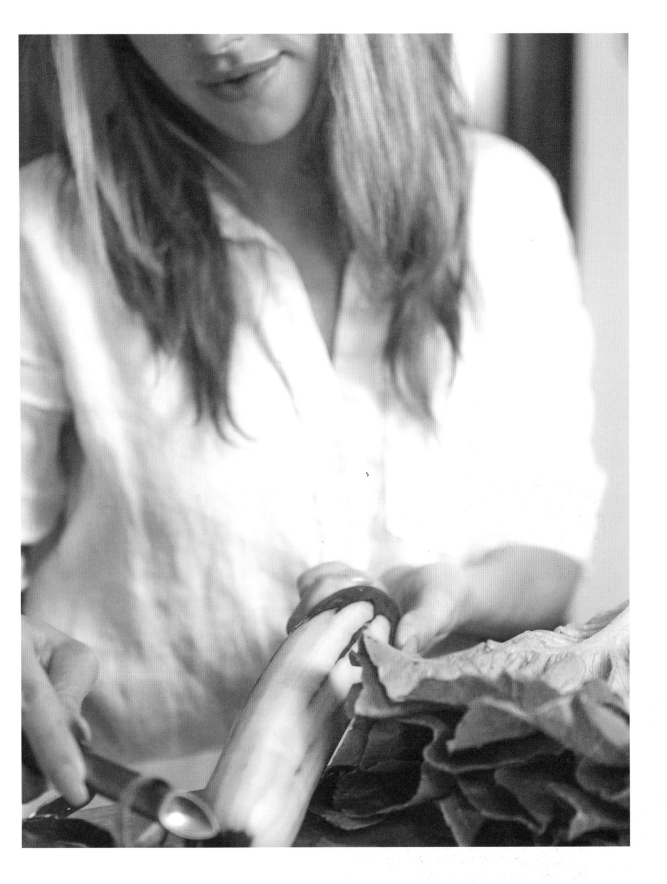

An Eat-Healthy-Anywhere Guide to Eating Out

The main reason eating out causes so many disturbances to our health is because we are not in control of what our food is made with or how it's prepared.

It's very important to know what kind of oil is in your food, how much salt and sugar have been added, and the source of the ingredients, which isn't easy when you aren't the master of your own food. The trick to ordering the right food while dining out is to be aware of which dishes will throw you out of balance.

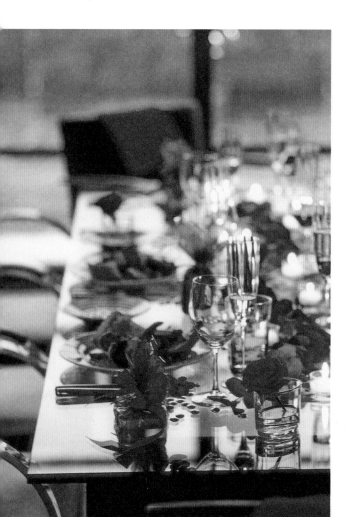

Generally, people go out to eat for a special occasion or celebration. If you are eating out daily, however, I highly suggest you make yourself a little more comfortable in the kitchen because one of the best tools you have for healing your body is your own ability to nourish yourself. When you are cooking, you are in complete conscious control of the food you are combining, the quality of the ingredients, and the love you put into the meal. Of course, we all want or need to eat out from time to time. Here are some suggestions to help you make the best choices.

Tips and Tricks for Eating Out

- **No food is ever off-limits:** You can choose any food you like as long as it is eaten in an appropriate quantity and with the proper precautions. Be honest with yourself and don't overindulge to the point that you are sick. Only you can know the appropriate amount of food for you. The best way to know is by listening to your body. As soon as you feel heavy, tired, or bloated, recognize that your body is telling you you've eaten too much food. To avoid these uncomfortable symptoms, take small bites, chew food fully, enjoy your food, breathe in and out between bites, and be conscious of how you are feeling. If you notice that you have eaten a significant amount of food but still feel hungry, allow yourself ten minutes to digest before

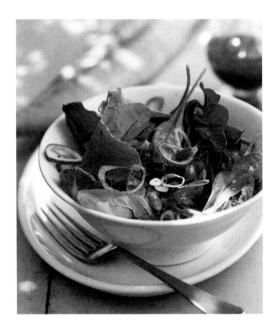

vinegar will also aid in fat metabolism by stimulating bile production.

- **Choose the right drinks:** Order hot water with lemon as soon as you arrive at a restaurant. Hot water is a great way to stoke your digestive fire and the sour taste of lemon improves digestion while detoxing your system. Drink hot water with lemon before your meal and only during the meal if you are really thirsty. Do not drink ice water or cool drinks because they will cause gas or bloating and put out your digestive fire.

- **Avoid perfectionism:** As always, don't be stressed out by too many guidelines. It will be difficult to find the perfect Ayurveda-approved meal on most menus. Be reasonable and just do what you can.

Further Suggestions to Dine Out with Ease

- Add a pinch of black pepper to a glass of warm water or to your food to help difficult-to-digest foods move through your system more easily.

- Eat the parsley that is used to garnish your food. It aids digestion and offers a bitter taste that will help move things downward.

- Don't be afraid to ask the waiter plenty of questions about the food. Get to know what you will be eating before ordering. And don't be afraid to ask whether they can adapt the way a dish is prepared or served. You may be worried that it will be annoying but the restaurant will have a whole kitchen full of food, so hopefully they can find a compromise.

- Favor simple meals made with just a few ingredients that are easy to digest. For example, choose a taco instead of a seven-layer burrito. Simpler meals conform to the rules of food combining.

ordering or eating more. Whatever you eat, take note of how you feel for future reference. Eating should be a joyous activity that leaves you feeling energized, vivacious, and strong.

- **Chew your food:** Whenever you are in the worst of food situations, chew your food carefully. Saliva has digestive enzymes that help to start breaking down the food before you even swallow. Try to "digest" the food as much as possible in your mouth. Unchewed food is very difficult to digest, especially if the food is raw or poorly combined.

- **Always order vegetable sides:** When eating out, vegetable sides are always a good choice—you could even consider having the sides as your main meal. If your meal is lacking fiber, order vegetable sides or incorporate a salad. The bitter taste of a salad will increase bile production and flush the gallbladder, helping you digest heavy fats. Order your salad with oil and vinegar on the side instead of with a creamy or heavy dressing. The sour taste of

- Avoid eating too much complimentary bread and butter; not only will it fill you up with empty calories but also it could leave you feeling bloated.
- If you are trying to lose weight or have a Kapha imbalance, minimize cream sauces, excessive amounts of cheese, carb-bombs, and too much salt.
- Reduce the amount of fried food you order–especially tortilla chips–because the oils they have been cooked in may be rancid, overheated, or of poor quality. It's especially important to avoid rancid oils or overcooked oils if you have a Pitta imbalance.
- Choose fish over meat, but only if the fish was caught in the wild. If you eat meat, select pasture-raised, grass-fed, and/or grass-finished meat. (What's the difference between grass-fed and grass-finished meat? Well, grass-finished cows eat nothing but grass their entire lives, whereas grass-fed cows are started on a grass diet and finished on a grain diet.) It's best only to eat organic, antibiotic-free, and/or hormone-free meat.
- Choose rice over pasta. Rice is easier to digest, and it is very grounding and nourishing to Vata. Wheat-based pasta dishes are heavier and tend to be combined with even heavier oily sauces.
- Soups are usually very easy to digest and tend to be full of fiber-packed vegetables. However, bear in mind that cream-based soups like clam chowders, lobster bisque, and broccoli and cheddar soup don't count.
- For dessert, choose a pie over cakes, ice-creams, or cheesecakes. Even though most pies are a bad food combination, they generally contain whole foods, fiber, and less sugar (although not by much).

Specific Tips for Your Dosha

VATA types should avoid raw food and beans.

PITTA should avoid fried, oily foods. You can always ask for some butter or olive oil on the side to fatten up your dish.

KAPHA should avoid wheat, dairy, and sugar.

THE BEST FOODS TO EAT OUT BY RESTAURANT TYPE

The following chart provides a handy guide to the best and worst foods to order when eating out, organized by type of restaurant. There is usually something available within any cuisine, as long as you choose carefully.

Restaurant	Best choices	Avoid
All-you-can-eat buffet	It's okay to take a small portion of any food you'd like to try from the buffet but make sure the majority of your meal is healthy (steamed or sautéed veggies) and try to choose the best possible food combinations. Eat slowly.	Heavy carbs, oily meats, and overcooked oily food.
Bar and pub	Salads, dairy-free soups, baked or mashed potatoes, and veggie side dishes.	Fried foods, cheeseburgers, and French onion soup.
BBQ restaurant	Salads, corn (sweetcorn), coleslaw, veggies, and baked potatoes.	Fried foods, such as wings and fries, and too much BBQ sauce (it has too much sugar).
Breakfast restaurant	Gluten-free toast (or whole-wheat toast if gluten-free toast is not an option), fresh fruit (eat on its own or before anything else), veggie omelets (no cheese), and oatmeal (porridge). You can always substitute salad for potatoes or toast.	Dishes that combine meat, eggs, cheese, and bread. Non-gluten-free pancakes, biscuits (scones) or pastries that have shortening in them, syrups and jams (especially those made with corn syrup), French toast (it is often made with refined white flour, which is carb heavy and nutritionally unbalanced), and donuts (they're deep fried and have no nutritional value).
Café	Soups and salads with oil and vinegar on the side.	Muffins, bagels, and carb-only meals (they contain little to no nutritional value and will be difficult to digest).
Chinese restaurant	Vegetable-based dishes (sometimes called "vegetable delight" on the menu) or mixed vegetables with rice.	Deep-fried dishes, sugar-rich sauces, dishes made with MSG.
Deli	Veggie and hummus wraps, pickles, three-bean salads, and other salads containing fiber.	Meatball sandwiches, Italian heroes (submarine sandwiches), cold cuts, sandwiches made with cured meats (which contain nitrates).

Restaurant	Best choices	Avoid
Gas station	To be honest, it's best you don't feed yourself where you feed your car. If you have to grab a snack on the road, make sure it's real food. The best option is always fruit if they have it. Try a banana, apple, or orange.	Slushies, hot dogs, candy bars, donuts, chips (crisps), muffins, protein bars containing no real food ingredients, and other junk-food options.
Indian restaurant	Dals, vegetarian dishes (ask for dishes without butter or cream sauces), salads. Add yogurt to cool down a dish with very hot spices.	Very spicy options, dishes with a lot of rice or potatoes together, creamy or very oily sauces, naan bread (because of the refined flour), fried dough balls, and overcooked buffet food (it is not often fresh).
Italian restaurant	Vegetable side dishes, fish with lemon sauce (ask for no butter or to substitute olive oil for butter), salads, pasta primavera, and minestrone soup.	Pasta dishes with cream or meat sauces, garlic bread, and cheesy dishes.
Japanese restaurant	Sushi, rice noodles, and soup (for a lighter option).	Teriyaki sauces that contain sugar and refined oils.
Mediterranean restaurant	Most things on the menu are good options.	Deep-fried foods like falafel (lentils/chickpeas are difficult to digest).
Mexican restaurant	Veggie or fish fajitas are best. Veggies tacos, salads, and guacamole.	Burritos with too many ingredients (burritos tend to have the worst food combinations and are belly bombs), tortilla chips (they may contain rancid oils and too much extra salt, which is aggravating to Pitta), cheese, sour cream. Some wheat tortillas have hydrogenated oils.
Pizza restaurant	Grandma slices (pizza with sauce and herbs only, no cheese–ask for cooked veggies on top), white pizzas with a green veggie on top, thin-crust pizzas, or salad slices. Always ask for a gluten-free option.	Pizzas with too much cheese and/or meat and deep-dish pizzas.
Thai restaurant	Most foods are good options–especially vegetable pad thai, noodles, and soups.	Avoid anything fried, and avoid soy, if possible, unless it's organic and non-genetically modified.
Vending machine	This should be an absolute last resort! If you must buy snacks from a vending machine, opt for a bag of nuts.	Candy bars, chips (crisps), snack cakes, and junk food that contains just sugar and gluten and has no substance.

How to Relieve Digestive Discomfort

If you have just eaten a large, poorly combined, and heavy meal, follow these tips to relieve yourself from discomfort.

- Take a gentle walk after the meal. Taking a short walk around the block will rev your metabolism, add an element of mobility, and break up heaviness from overeating. Don't go for a run (especially if you are of Pitta constitution)–the aim is to get things moving in a downward flow, not to sweat out any toxins you've just eaten. You can save your sweat for a day later.
- I recommend triphala (see page 156) to most of my clients. It is an herbal formula that is balancing to all three doshas. It is a natural, rejuvenating detoxifier and purifier that is good to take nightly and it can also be handy to take when you have overindulged. Triphala is made of three rasayana (nourishing support) herbs: amalaka, bibhitaki, and haritaki. It promotes healthy weight loss and steady agni and it also tones, nourishes, and strengthens the entire body. If taken after a meal, triphala will give your body a gentle cleanse, help remove any lingering toxicity formed by the food, and reset your digestion so you feel ready to go the next day.
- The mindset you are in while eating will affect the way you digest, process, and absorb your food. It's important to remember not to feel guilty or regret the things that you do. You can't change the past, only look toward the future for another chance to change. If eating certain food makes you feel awful, you'll inevitably learn that it's not in alignment with you to eat that food. However, it won't ruin your progress if you decide to eat a cheeseburger, cake, burrito, pizza, etc. once in a while. Focus on the good. Give thanks to your body, release guilt, and never regret. Life is about living and having fun so don't beat yourself up over the small stuff … especially food. Focus on being thankful, enjoy the quality of the time you have with loved ones, and don't worry about the food.

Overleaf are simplified versions of ancient Ayurvedic tricks that will relieve digestive discomfort and help you stay balanced.

WARM WATER WITH FRESH LEMON JUICE

This should be drunk first thing in the morning (see page 149) to cleanse your bowels, promote digestion, and remove toxins. If you are following the 7-Day Meal Plan for Vata (see pages 110–111), make the recipe as below, adding a grated ½-inch (1-cm) piece of fresh ginger to the water in the saucepan before heating. If you are following the 7-Day Meal Plan for Kapha (see pages 112–113), make the recipe as below, adding 1 teaspoon raw honey to the finished drink when it has cooled to a warm temperature (see page 99).

1 lemon

1½–3¾ cups (350–900 ml) water

Serves 1

Wash the lemon and then either juice half of it or cut the lemon in half and squeeze some juice into a large mug. Add the rest of the lemon to the mug. Heat the water in a small saucepan on the stove until you see little bubbles forming at the bottom of the pan–do not let the water boil. Pour the warm water into the mug with the lemon juice.

Alternatively, if you don't have access to a stovetop, feel free to use a microwave. Heat the water in a microwave-safe cup (ceramic is preferred) in 30-second increments. Heating the water in a microwave for 40–50 seconds will usually warm the water to an enjoyable temperature.

AMA GUT FLUSH

This recipe stimulates digestive fire (agni), flushes toxins, and keeps ama at bay. It will be particularly helpful for Vata and Kapha. Pittas should almost never use this remedy and should instead drink Warm Water with Fresh Lemon Juice (see left), unless otherwise advised by a specialist. Yes, the Ama Gut Flush is that potent, and you don't want to cause more imbalances in the body.

For convenience, you can make this mixture at the beginning of the week and store it in a jar in the refrigerator. Take a shot prior to each meal or add it to a glass of warm water.

2 cups (475 ml) water

2-inch (5-cm) piece of fresh ginger, peeled and grated

juice of 2 lemons

2 teaspoons Himalayan pink salt

Serves 2

Put the water in a saucepan and bring to a boil. Add the remaining ingredients. Once the water returns to a boil, remove from the heat, cover, and let stand for 2 hours.

Using a strainer or cheesecloth (muslin), strain the liquid into a jar and store for up to 1 week in the refrigerator.

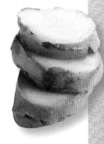

CELERY JUICE ELIXIR

Drinking celery juice on an empty stomach helps to produce the stomach acid HCL, which breaks down proteins in the gut, restores electrolyte balance, detoxes the liver and kidneys, hydrates the skin, and lowers blood pressure. Celery is also an excellent source of natural sodium, which can help beat salty cravings when consumed daily. This elixir is suitable for all three doshas.

1 bunch of celery, chopped

1 lemon, halved and peeled

Serves 1

Juice the celery and lemon. Alternatively, if you don't have a juicer, put the celery and lemon in a food processor or blender and blend on a high speed until well blended, then use a nut bag or cheesecloth (muslin) to strain the juice. Drink on an empty stomach for most benefits. The elixir will keep for up to 2 days in an airtight container or jar in the refrigerator.

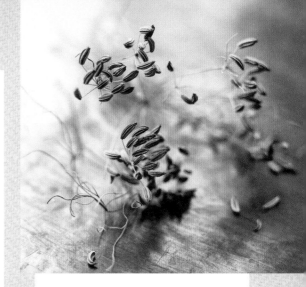

THE FENNEL TRICK

At one time or another, most of us have eaten too much in one meal and instantly felt bloated. That's okay. Remember, this is a lifelong journey and lapses are bound to happen at some point. Luckily, there is an easy fix for a stuffed and bloated tummy: Fennel. One of the simplest ways to incorporate it into your diet is to chew about twenty fennel seeds after a meal. Fennel helps to digest heavy sauces and carb-centric dishes, which is why you see a bowl of fennel seeds at the exit of most Indian restaurants. Drinking warm water will also help lessen the bloat.

CUT SUGAR CRAVINGS

Cardamom is one of those beautiful spices that is used throughout this book. If you happen to crave sweet things frequently, specifically after eating a savory meal, chew on fresh cardamom seeds. This may sound strange but it actually works– it calms the nerves in the brain and diminishes the craving for something sweet.

MODERN KITCHARI RESET

Sometimes we can overload our system and no remedy seems to help. Kitchari is a tool I fall back on when my body needs a rest, the change of season has me feeling out of balance, or I simply need to cleanse and reset. It can help give your digestive system a break and reset your body back to balance. It is an easy-to-digest complete food that balances all three doshas (hence why it's so powerful). Kitchari can be eaten every day if you enjoy it. If liked, you can serve this dish topped with your favorite steamed veggies.

2 tablespoons coconut oil

1½ teaspoons cumin seeds

1½ teaspoons fennel seeds

½ teaspoon fenugreek seeds

¼ teaspoon black mustard seeds

1½ teaspoons ground coriander

1 tablespoon minced fresh ginger

½ teaspoon turmeric powder

pinch of asafetida (hing)

4 cups (950 ml) vegetable stock or water

½ cup (100 g) split yellow mung beans, soaked overnight in a bowl of purified water and then drained and rinsed

½ cup (85 g) sprouted quinoa, rinsed

1-inch (2.5-cm) strip of kombu

sea salt

TO GARNISH

½ cup (25 g) chopped cilantro (fresh coriander)

1 lime, cut into wedges

Serves 4

Heat the coconut oil in a heavy-bottomed saucepan over a medium heat, then add the cumin, fennel, fenugreek, and mustard seeds and cook for a few minutes to release the aromatics, until the mustard seeds start to pop. Add the remaining spices and stir to combine. Add 1 cup (250 ml) of the vegetable stock or water, followed by the mung beans, quinoa, and kombu, then add the remainder of the stock or water. Cover and bring to a boil, then reduce the heat to a simmer and cook for 40 minutes or until the beans and quinoa are tender and the mixture has thickened to a porridge consistency, checking from time to time to make sure the quinoa does not stick to the bottom of the pan. Season with salt. (If you prefer a soupier consistency, add some extra water and simmer for longer to get a thicker stew.)

Divide the kitchari between bowls and garnish with cilantro (fresh coriander) and lime wedges to squeeze over. The kitchari will keep for up to 4 days in an airtight container in the refrigerator.

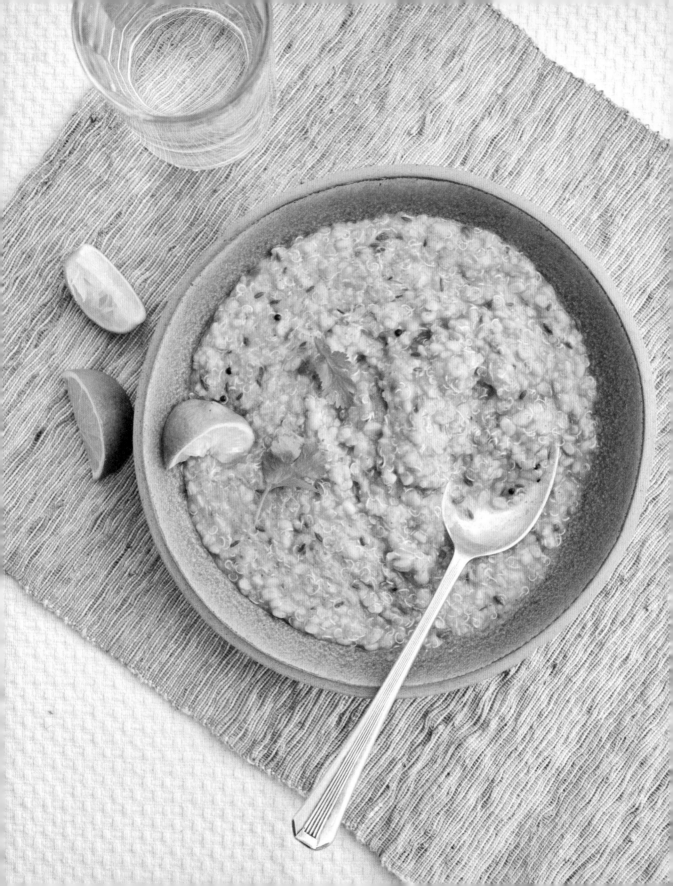

When we turn to the wisdom of nature to cure our pains, we are taking action instead of depending on drugs. All it takes is one step in the natural direction to set you on the path. All you need is one habit to be the catalyst for them all. Begin to bring awareness into your life. Take small steps back toward nature. All the answers are in front of you, all the power is inside of you.

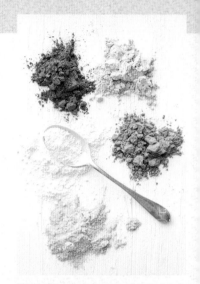

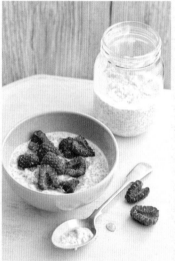

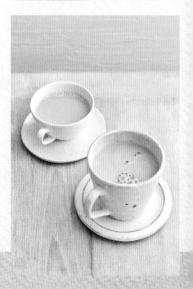

chapter 3

RECIPES: EAT AND DRINK FOR YOUR DOSHA

In this chapter, I share with you the recipes I prescribe to my clients and follow myself. I have included sweet and savory dishes that everyone can feel good about indulging in. To help you transition into a more wholesome lifestyle, you will find my recommendations for the best brands currently on the market in the Resources (see page 156).

Choosing Ingredients

Here are a few simple things to keep in mind when you choose the ingredients for the recipes in this book:

- When choosing ingredients (including spices), select organic whenever possible.
- Pasture-raised and pastured eggs differ from other eggs on the market because the hens roam free, eating plants, insects, and organic feed. The labels "organic," "cage-free," and "free-range" don't necessarily mean that the living environment for the hens was safe or open.
- Use purified (filtered) water. You can buy purified water or install a water filter in your home. If possible, avoid using water from the faucet (tap), as this contains cancer-causing chemicals, and deionized distilled water, which has had its essential minerals removed during the manufacturing process.
- Choose nut milks without stabilizers or, more importantly, carrageenan (a food additive that can cause inflammation of the intestines).

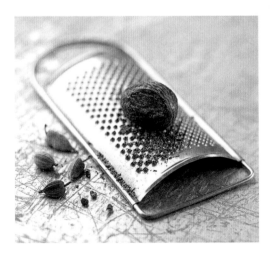

Herbs and Spices

Did you know that you probably have life-changing medicine in your own home? The pantry is often overlooked when it comes to medicinal healing herbs. Utilizing the power of herbs is a wonderful way of incorporating the methods of Ayurveda and self-love into your life. If you don't stock your spice rack with these herbs and spices already, I guarantee they will soon become a staple in your everyday cooking.

You can sneak herbs and spices into virtually any type of food or drink you make, instantly boosting their nutritional benefits. Here are a few of my recommendations for herbs and spices to enhance digestion and metabolism, prevent digestive disorders, and cleanse toxins (ama) from the body: asafetida (also known as hing), black pepper, cardamom, cayenne pepper, cinnamon, coriander, cumin, fennel, fenugreek, ginger, manjistha powder, mint, mustard seeds, nutmeg, rosemary, turmeric, and dried chamomile, lavender, and rose flowers.

Adaptogens

Adaptogens are herbs, superfoods, and other substances that have nonspecific actions on the body, meaning they support all the major systems as well as regulatory functions. They don't harm or cause additional stress to the body. Instead, they help the body adapt to many and varied environmental and physiological stresses, and they should be included in our diets to enhance and protect our immune and hormonal systems.

Mucuna Pruriens

Mucuna pruriens (also known as kapikachhu) is a legume that contains L-dopa, which is an amino acid found in the body that transforms into dopamine in the brain. Dopamine is a neurotransmitter that allows the dynamic functioning of the brain. Higher levels of dopamine can help with sleep, brain function, and an expanded sense of well-being. Mucuna pruriens is known for its ability to lift moods and enhance sexual function. You can use it in a sleep or energy tonic and it will work naturally for what your body needs most.

Amalaki

Amalaki (or amla for short) is one of my all-time favorite adaptogens. I love the way it tastes and smells, and it's the ultimate beauty food. Amla nourishes the blood, detoxes and restores health to the liver, is rich in vitamin C, and is known as the immortality fruit. It can be purchased as both a herb and a powder, but I recommend using the powder for tonics. I add amla powder to all of my food. People ask me what I do to achieve glowing skin and amla is definitely a factor.

Astragalus

Astragalus is an Ayurvedic root (bought as a powder) that is used to balance hormones, specifically cortisol levels. You'll find many popular herbal formulas contain astragalus nowadays because of the rise in people's stress levels. Astragalus helps balance those suffering from chronic fatigue, immune disorders, kidney disease, and high blood pressure.

Lucuma

Lucuma powder is derived from the lucuma fruit. It is rich in vitamin B3, beta carotene, calcium, protein, iron, and zinc. Lucuma powder tastes similar to maple syrup but is lower on the glycemic index.

Maca

Maca is an adaptogenic root that helps to balance hormones, promote energy and stamina, and boost memory, and is additionally rich in essential vitamins and minerals.

Medicinal Mushrooms

Medicinal mushrooms have become widely used for multiple reasons. They help to rebuild the immune system, protect the body from disease, are rich in minerals, provide energy, fight inflammation, and reduce stress. The main mushrooms you need to know about are chaga, reishi, he shou wu, and cordyceps.

Rhodiola

Rhodiola is considered an adaptogenic flower that helps greatly to combat the effects of stress. Along with proper diet, exercise, and care, rhodiola can help ease symptoms of stress, depression, and anxiety and boosts cognitive function. Rhodiola contains essential chemical compounds that help reduce and maintain healthy cortisol levels. Rosavin, a compound found in rhodiola, is responsible for assisting in reducing visceral body fat. It's important to use a high-quality form of rhodiola because where it is sourced from can make a difference to whether its chemical compounds are intact or not. (See page 156 for recommended brands.)

Pearl Powder

As you can see, most of the adaptogens can beautify and balance the body. One adaptogen that is not found in Ayurvedic medicine, but rather in Chinese medicine, is pearl powder. Pearl powder is simply crushed pearls. Taking this adaptogen internally can boost collagen production and increase cellular turnover. Pearls are rich in calcium, which strengthens hair, teeth, and nails. I take pearl powder internally in tonics but use it in my homemade skin care as well. Pearl powder for use in recipes should be labeled as food grade, but it sometimes isn't. However, you can use most pearl powder internally the same as externally, provided that it is pure and there is no filler in the powder (which would be listed under the ingredients).

Ashwagandha

Ashwagandha is an adaptogenic herb that has been used for centuries to enhance youthfulness and reproductive function and nourish supple skin, lustrous shiny hair, and the internal organs for an all-over body glow. Ashwagandha is also known for its plethora of important minerals, including magnesium, which is a crucial mineral in the body that can help to soothe anxiety, alleviate depression, improve sleep, and has a calming effect on the body's physiological and nervous systems. Among many other great qualities, ashwagandha increases nitric oxide in the body, which is why it's known for its aphrodisiac qualities.

The incredible thing about adaptogens is their multifunctional qualities. Not only does ashwagandha soothe the nervous system but it deeply energizes the body (although it's not a stimulant), balances hormones, and supports healthy adrenals.

Moringa

Moringa is one of those miracle herbs that can be used for many ailments (like most adaptogens). Moringa slows the effects of aging, balances hormones, improves digestion, is rich in micronutrients, balances blood sugar levels, and is rich in protein. I love to use moringa in smoothies but it also makes for an amazing face mask (see page 139) because it's packed with free-radical fighting antioxidants.

Schizandra Berry

Schizandra berry is a beauty adaptogen that focuses on the adrenals, liver, skin, and hormones. This beautifully tart berry increases libido, improves mental function, reduces inflammation, cleanses the liver, aids stomach-related imbalances, and improves the body's ability to deal with stress. I like to add schizandra powder to pancakes, tonics, smoothies, and raw chocolate for an overall beautifying effect.

Pine Pollen

Pine pollen powder has a powerful androgenic effect on the body, especially in men. Pine pollen has the ability to increase DHEA (a hormone produced by the adrenal glands) and testosterone levels, making this a virility-boosting adaptogen. Women may take it too for low libido and hormone imbalance. When taken over a long period of time, like most adaptogens, you may feel increased strength, stamina, and sexual health. The combination of schizandra berry and pine pollen makes for a perfect sex tonic.

From top to bottom: pine pollen, ashwagandha, moringa, schizandra berry, and pearl powder.

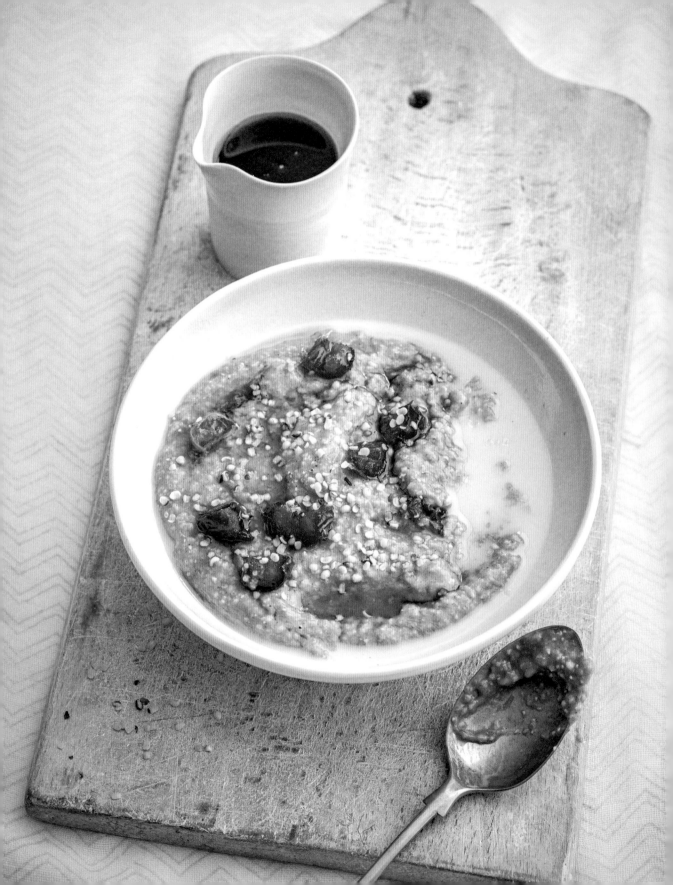

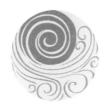

RECIPES FOR VATA

Vatas function best when they eat at predictable meal times to keep digestion regular. If you have a predominantly Vata constitution, you should favor well-cooked foods including vegetables, and fruit. Increasing your healthy fat intake will aid in lubricating dryness in the body, so try to add ghee or cold-pressed olive oil to every meal. Use warming spices such as ginger, cinnamon, cumin, coriander, and black pepper. Avoid cold, raw, or frozen foods because the coolness of these foods can cause digestive distress for Vata. Drink warm water or tea throughout the day.

BREAKFAST Vata Breakfast Bowl

This simple breakfast dish contains the perfect balance of nutrients to nourish and fuel Vata.

1 teaspoon ghee or coconut oil

1 teaspoon ground cinnamon

1 teaspoon ground cardamom

1 teaspoon ground ginger

2–3 cups (475–700 ml) water

⅔ cup (60 g) gluten-free oat bran

⅓ cup (75 ml) almond milk

½ teaspoon maple syrup

2 Medjool dates, chopped

1 tablespoon hemp seeds (optional)

Serves 1

Heat the ghee or oil and spices in a saucepan over a medium heat. Add the water and oat bran and cook for 5 minutes (or according to instructions on the oat bran packet), stirring continuously, until the oats soften and thicken to a porridge consistency. Pour into a bowl and top with the milk, maple syrup, dates, and hemp seeds, if using.

MAIN Cauliflower Tikka Masala

This is my go-to recipe for chilly nights. It is an easy way to add warming spices and healthy fats into your diet.

1 tablespoon ghee

½ teaspoon mustard seeds

½-inch (1-cm) piece of fresh ginger, peeled and finely grated

6 garlic cloves, minced

1½ cups (175 g) diced white onion (about 1 onion)

¾ cup (175 ml) full-fat coconut milk

¾ teaspoon garam masala

½ teaspoon ground coriander

¼ teaspoon ground turmeric

½ teaspoon ground cinnamon

½ teaspoon sea salt

1 cauliflower, cut into medium-small florets

freshly chopped cilantro (fresh coriander), to garnish

Serves 2

Heat the ghee in a large sauté pan over a medium heat. Add the mustard seeds and cook for 30 seconds (until they sizzle and pop), then immediately add the ginger, garlic, and onion and cook for a few minutes, stirring frequently, until fragrant and the onion starts to become translucent.

Put the coconut milk in a food processor or blender, add the onion mixture, and blend on high until smooth.

Pour the sauce into the sauté pan, add the remaining spices and the salt and cauliflower, and toss well to coat the cauliflower with the sauce. Cover and cook over a low heat for about 10 minutes or until the cauliflower is tender. Serve garnished with cilantro (fresh coriander). Any leftovers will keep for up to 3 days in an airtight container in the refrigerator.

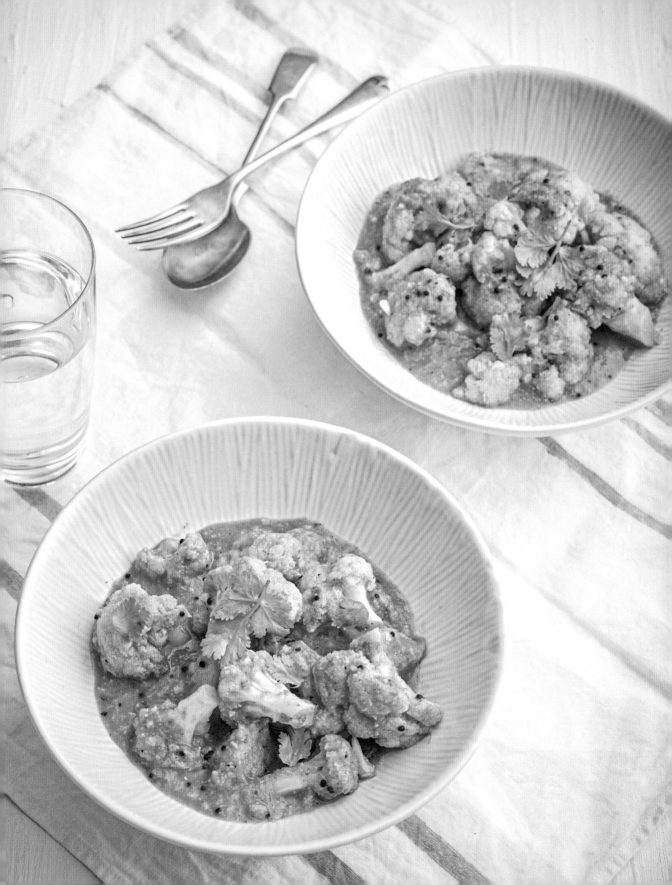

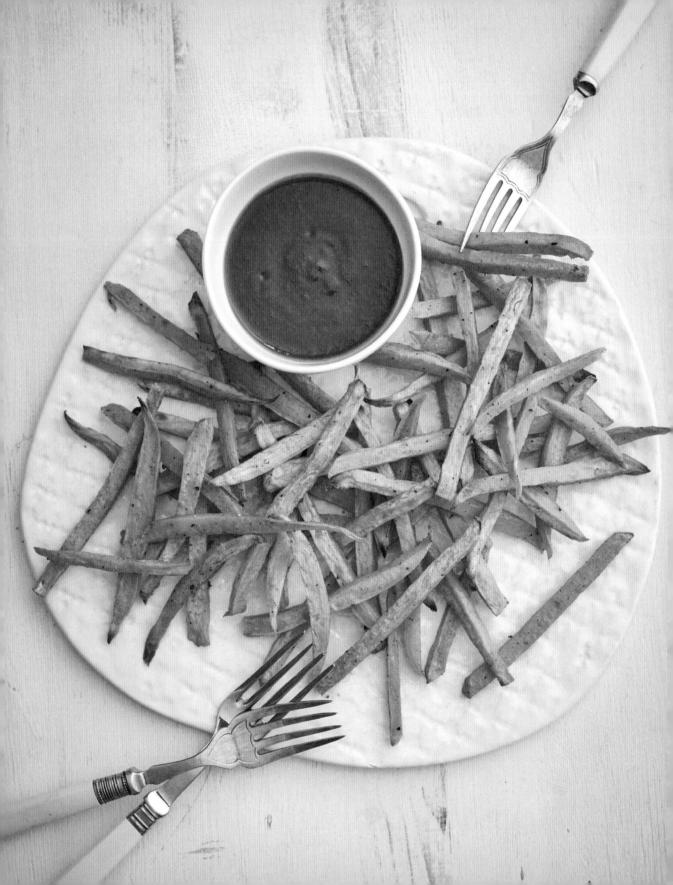

SNACK Spiced Sweet Potato Fries

Enjoy these fries as a snack with hummus (such as the Cucumber and Dill Hummus on page 72) or sugar-free ketchup.

2 tablespoons cold-pressed olive oil

⅛ teaspoon sea salt

⅛ teaspoon ground black pepper

⅛ teaspoon ground cumin

⅛ teaspoon ground coriander

⅛ teaspoon ground cinnamon

2 lb (900 g) sweet potatoes, peeled and cut into ¼-inch (5-mm) fries

Preheat the oven to 250°F/120°C/Gas ½.

In a large bowl, combine all the ingredients except the sweet potatoes. Add the sweet potatoes and toss to coat them with the spiced oil mixture.

Spread out the sweet potatoes in a single layer on a nonstick baking sheet and bake in the oven for 30 minutes, turning occasionally, until lightly browned. Remove from the oven and let cool a little before eating. Any leftovers will keep for up to 3 days in an airtight container in the refrigerator.

Serves 2

SMOOTHIE Chris's Travel Shake

My dad, Chris, is quite the world traveler and he has taken me and my family along for the ride on many of his journeys. This smoothie is an ode to my Abu (which means "father" in Arabic), because Vata needs extra nourishment when traveling. The ginger, fennel, and dates help to ground Vata both before and after travel.

1 cup (250 ml) unsweetened almond milk

½ teaspoon ground cinnamon, plus extra to decorate

⅛-inch (3-mm) piece of peeled fresh ginger

½ teaspoon ground fennel seeds

1 teaspoon ghee or coconut butter

2 large Medjool dates, pitted

Serves 1

Combine all the ingredients in a food processor or blender and blend on high until smooth. Pour into a glass or travel drink container and decorate with a sprinkling of cinnamon.

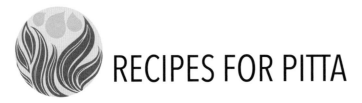

RECIPES FOR PITTA

Pittas function best when they eat several small meals throughout the day rather than just two or three big meals. If you have a predominantly Pitta constitution, favor cooling foods such as salads, steamed vegetables, fresh fruit, grains, and coconut milk. Pitta is very sensitive to chemical preservatives and artificial additives so be conscious of the products you buy. Avoid hot or spicy foods, fried food, sour food, tomatoes, vinegar, and yogurt. Spice-up your food with anti-inflammatory and cooling herbs and spices such as turmeric, mint, cilantro (fresh coriander), fennel seeds, parsley, and saffron. Drink room temperature cucumber-infused water throughout the day.

BREAKFAST Beauty Breakfast Pudding

The coconut and rose waters in this recipe are the perfect ingredients to cool Pittas. Prepare this dish the night before and you will have a satisfying breakfast by morning.

¾ cup (175 ml) full-fat coconut milk

½ teaspoon rose water

½ cup (120 ml) coconut water

¼ teaspoon sea salt

1 teaspoon pure vanilla extract or powder

¼ cup (20 g) unsweetened shredded coconut

¼ cup (40 g) chia seeds

½ cup (75 g) fresh raspberries

Serves 2

In an 8-oz (250-ml) mason jar, add all the ingredients except the raspberries and mix well. Close the jar and place in the refrigerator overnight or for 12 hours. To serve, scoop the pudding into bowls and top with the raspberries. Any leftovers will keep for up to 3 days in an airtight container in the refrigerator.

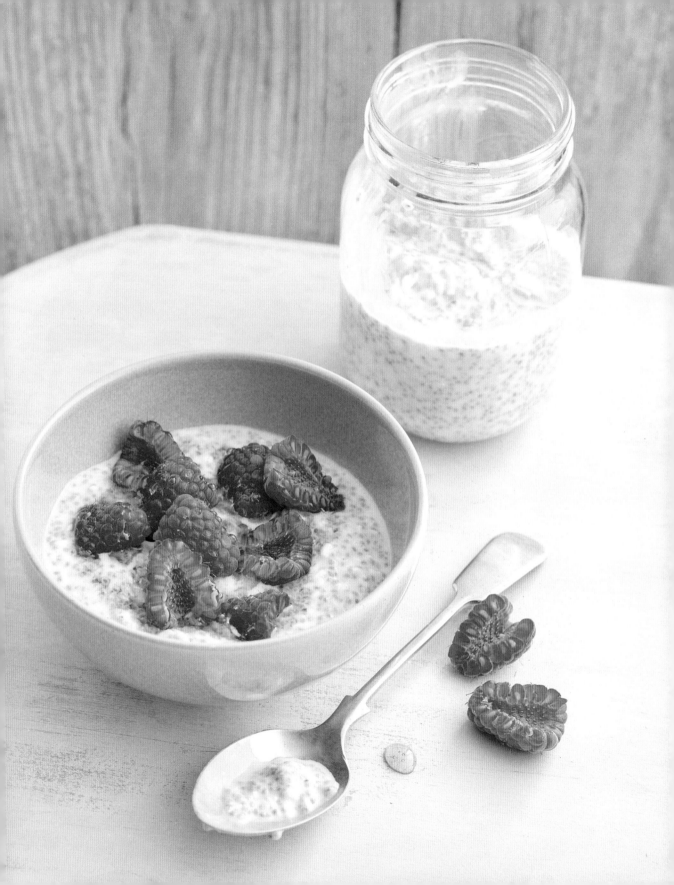

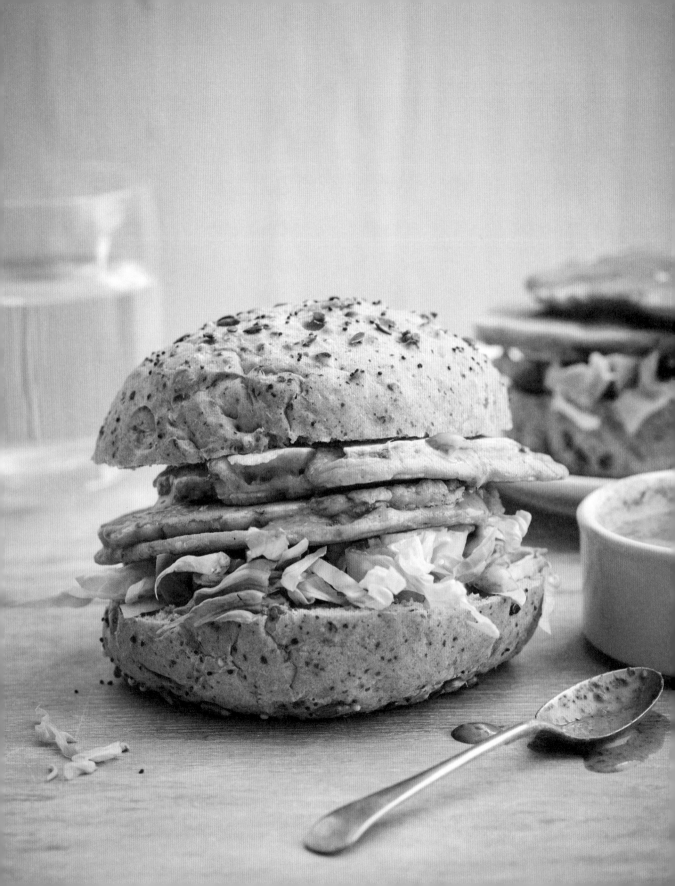

MAIN Turmeric Patty Sandwich with Mint and Cilantro Dressing

These protein-packed patties are anti-inflammatory, grain free, and easy to snack on. The dressing can also be used on salads or as a dip.

FOR THE PATTIES

3 pinches of sea salt

3 pinches of ground black pepper

½ teaspoon ground fennel seeds

½ teaspoon ground ginger

1 teaspoon ground turmeric

1 cup (90 g) sprouted chickpea flour

1 egg

1 cup (250 ml) sparkling mineral water

1 green (spring) onion, chopped

2 tablespoons chopped cilantro (fresh coriander)

1 teaspoon coconut oil, for greasing

FOR THE MINT AND CILANTRO DRESSING

1 large bunch of cilantro (fresh coriander)

2 tablespoons apple cider vinegar

1½ tablespoons chopped mint

½ cup (120 ml) full-fat coconut milk

1 teaspoon sea salt

TO SERVE

2 gluten-free buns, split in half

shredded lettuce

Serves 2

In a bowl, mix together the salt, pepper, fennel, ginger, turmeric, flour, and egg. Add the water and stir until combined, then gently fold the onion and cilantro (fresh coriander) into the batter.

Heat a nonstick or cast iron skillet (frying pan) over a medium heat. Dip a scrunched-up piece of kitchen paper into the oil and carefully use this to grease the hot skillet. Drop one quarter of the batter into the skillet and cook for 3–5 minutes, until you see little bubbles forming on the surface of the patty and the underside is golden brown. Flip over the patty and cook for a further 3–5 minutes. Keep the patties warm while you cook the remaining batter, greasing the pan with a little more oil if necessary.

To make the dressing, combine all the ingredients in a food processor or blender and blend on high until completely smooth.

To serve, arrange some lettuce on top of the base of each bun, then add 2 patties to each bun, drizzle over some of the dressing, and finish with the top of the buns. Any leftover dressing will keep for up to 3 days in an airtight container or glass jar in the refrigerator.

SNACK Cucumber and Dill Hummus

This is a great way to incorporate the cooling energetics of cucumber into any Pitta's diet.

2 cups (280 g) canned chickpeas, rinsed and drained

2 sprigs of dill

½ cucumber

½ teaspoon sea salt

2 tablespoons lemon juice

1 tablespoon cold-pressed olive oil, plus extra to serve

2 teaspoons tahini

TO SERVE

cucumber, cut into thin batons

carrot, cut into thin batons

celery stalks, cut into thin batons

Serves 2-3

Combine all the ingredients in a food processor or blender and pulse until smooth, scraping down the sides if needed.

Transfer the hummus to a bowl, drizzle with a little extra oil and serve with cucumber, carrot, and celery sticks. The hummus will keep for up to 1 week in an airtight container or jar in the refrigerator.

SMOOTHIE Logan's Tropical Smoothie

My brother, Logan, has always had a love for tropical fruits and tropical climates (he's my Pitta counterpart). He lives in Thailand among billowing trees lush with bananas and coconuts. This smoothie was inspired by my visit to his home. It is perfect for cooling Pitta's fiery energy and is sure to keep you satiated with healthy fiber.

1 large banana, peeled and chopped

½ cup (120 ml) half-fat coconut milk

juice of 1 lime

½ teaspoon ground cardamom

½ teaspoon ground turmeric

Serves 1

Combine all the ingredients in a food processor or blender and blend until smooth. Pour into a glass and enjoy!

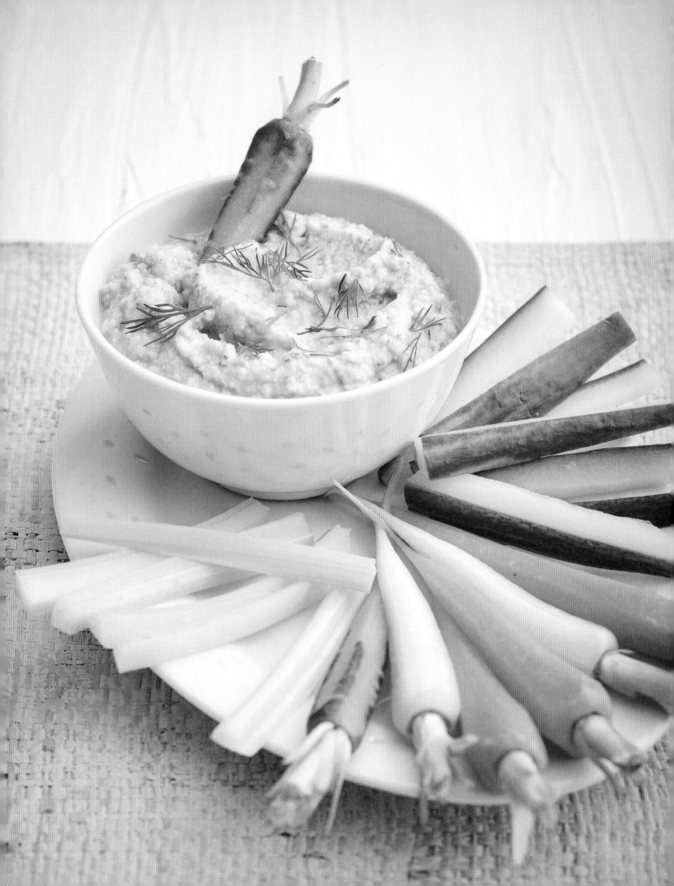

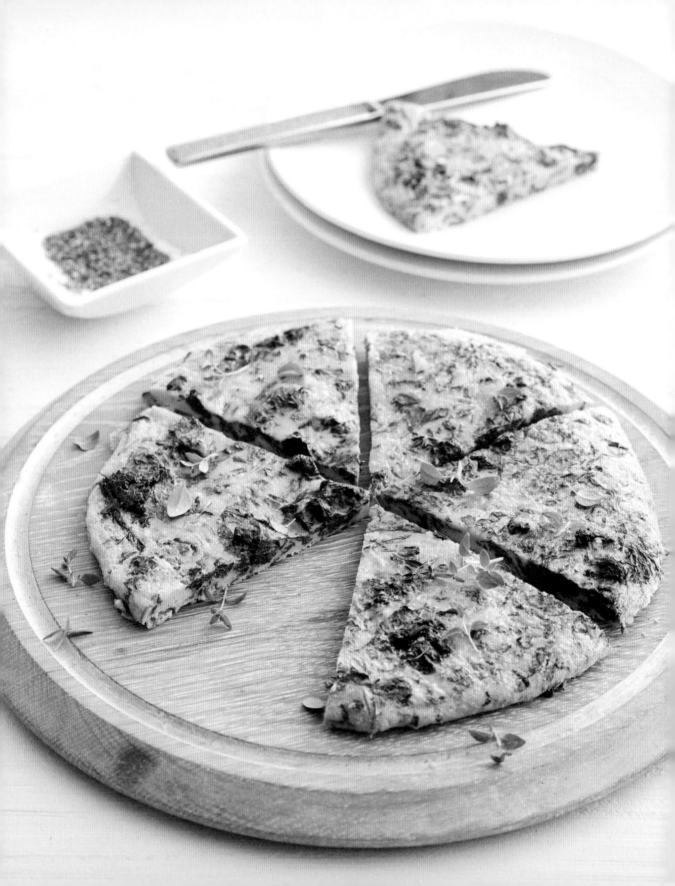

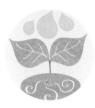

RECIPES FOR KAPHA

Kaphas function best when they avoid snacking and overeating and stick to two to three meals per day. This helps to not overload their slow-moving digestive system. If you have a predominantly Kapha constitution, you should favor light spicy foods such as non-creamy soups, steamed vegetables, fruits, leafy greens, raw nuts, and salads with minimum dressing. Spice-up your food with heating dry spices such as ginger, black pepper, mustard seeds, hingvastak (an Ayurvedic mix of herbs and spices), cinnamon, cloves, and basil.

BREAKFAST Spring Herbed Frittata

The bitter greens in this recipe help to balance and flush out the excess water in Kapha.

2 cups (120 g) chopped spinach

1⅔ cups (50 g) baby kale

6 eggs

1 teaspoon chopped parsley

1 teaspoon chopped thyme

1 teaspoon chopped basil

¼ teaspoon sea salt

¼ teaspoon ground black pepper

¼ teaspoon ghee or coconut oil

Serves 2

Preheat the oven to 350°F/180°C/Gas 4.

Cook the spinach and kale in a skillet (frying pan) over a high heat for 5 minutes or until the leaves have wilted and the excess water from the greens has boiled off.

In a large bowl, whip the eggs vigorously until fluffy, then gently fold in the herbs, salt, pepper, kale, and spinach.

Grease an ovenproof cast-iron skillet with ghee or coconut oil and place over a high heat for 3 minutes. Pour the egg mixture into the skillet and place in the oven. Bake for 20 minutes or until golden brown and set. Cut into slices and serve. Any leftover frittata will keep for up to 3 days in an airtight container in the refrigerator.

MAIN Lemon and Thyme Potatoes with Mixed Salad Greens

This bright, invigorating, and light potato recipe won't weigh Kapha down.

4 potatoes, peeled and cut into chunks

3 pinches of sea salt

1 bay leaf

4 pinches of ground black pepper

1 tablespoon ghee

1 teaspoon fresh thyme

juice of ½ lemon

mixed salad greens, to serve

Serves 2-3

Put 1 cup (250 ml) water in a large saucepan with a steamer basket and bring to the boil. Put the potatoes, salt, bay leaf, and black pepper into the basket, cover, and steam for 20 minutes or until the potatoes are tender. Discard the bay leaf.

Heat the ghee in a sauté pan, add the steamed potatoes and cook over a medium heat for 3 minutes, stirring occasionally, or until they begin to brown. Remove from heat, add the thyme and lemon juice and mix gently. Serve the potatoes on a bed of mixed salad greens. Any leftovers will keep for up to 3 days in an airtight container in the refrigerator.

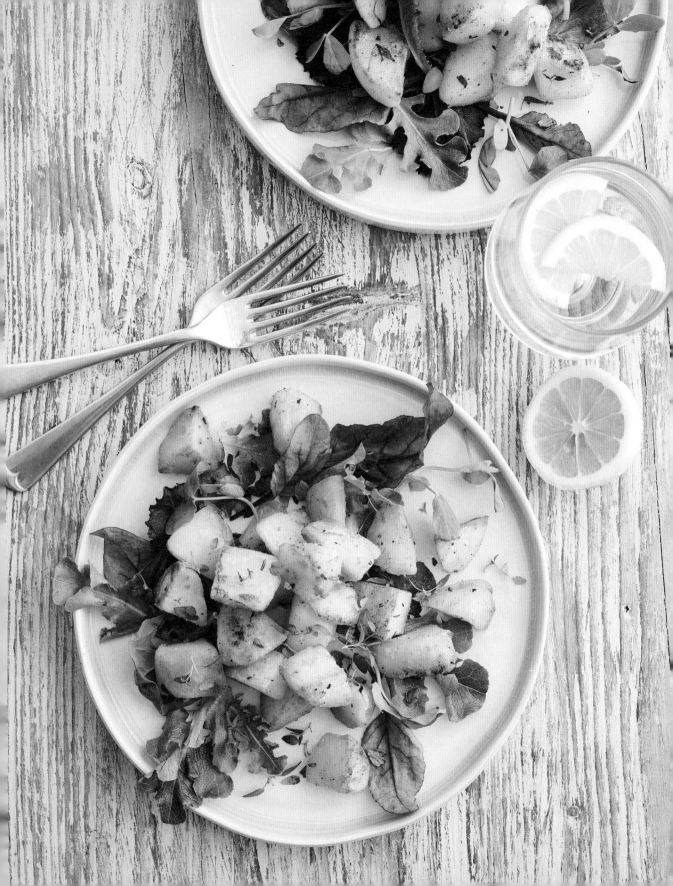

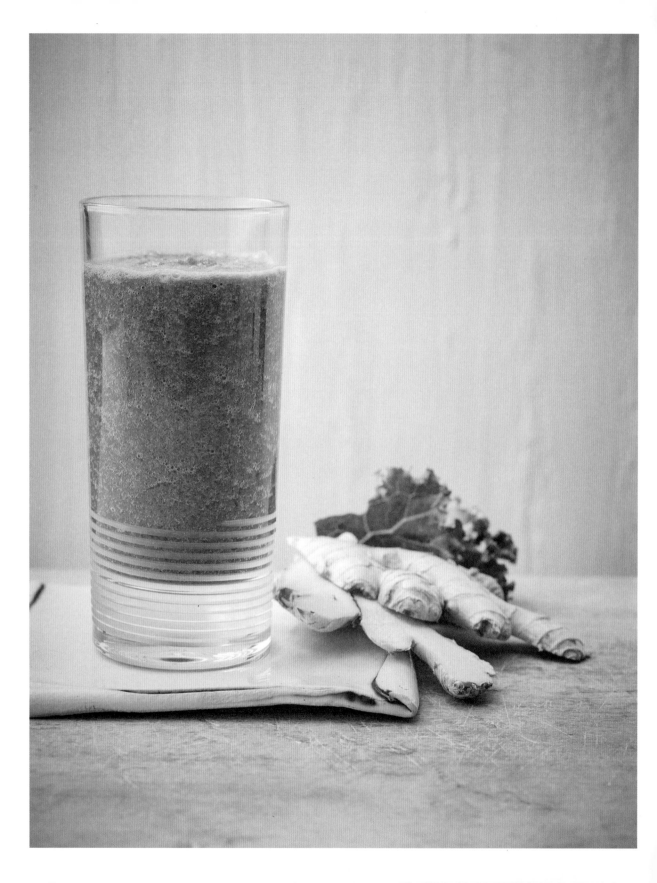

SNACK Beautifying Guacamole

This easy guacamole recipe is special because it contains half the fat of regular guacamole, making it easier for Kapha to digest and enjoy. Serve it over mixed salad greens or with grain-free chips (crisps) or crackers.

½ cup (70 g) diced avocado

1 cup (175 g) diced and steamed asparagus

juice of ½ lime

½ cup (60 g) chopped red onion

¼ teaspoon sea salt

2 teaspoons ground cumin

½ teaspoon ground black pepper

Serves 4

Combine all the ingredients in a food processor or blender and blend until smooth. The guacamole will keep for up to 2 days in an airtight container or jar in the refrigerator.

SMOOTHIE Lala's Detox Smoothie

My mom, Laurette (Lala for short), has always had a bad habit of skipping breakfast, until I introduced her to this gentle detox smoothie. Now, without missing a beat, she has it every morning before her cup of coffee. This combination of ginger, lemon, apple, and kale helps to detox and gently move Kapha along.

2-inch (5-cm) piece of fresh ginger, peeled

juice of 1 lemon

2 Granny Smith apples, halved and cored

2 cups (140 g) kale, chopped

1½ cups (350 ml) water

Serves 1

Combine all the ingredients in a food processor or blender and blend on high speed until smooth. Pour into a tall glass and serve immediately.

RECIPES FOR ALL THREE DOSHAS

Depending on how we pair food, our meals can balance us even if we are eating things that may not be suitable for our dosha. The following recipes can be tweaked and customized to your mind-body type. You can prepare them ahead of time and store them in the refrigerator for up to 5 days. When you are ready to eat, simply reheat the dish in the oven, on the stove, in the microwave, or enjoy it at room temperature.

Quinoa Bowl with Veggies

This quick lunch or dinner recipe is easy to make. It is great for digestion and a good solution for those who have little time to make their meals. There are three different options for the veggies, oils, and spices, so choose the right one for your dosha.

FOR THE QUINOA

¾ cup (130 g) sprouted quinoa, rinsed

1½ cups (350 ml) vegetable broth

FOR VATA

2 cups (250 g) chopped zucchini (courgette)

1 tablespoon ghee

½ teaspoon ground ginger

pinch of sea salt

FOR PITTA

2 cups (150 g) cauliflower florets

1 tablespoon coconut oil

½ teaspoon ground turmeric

pinch of sea salt

FOR KAPHA

2 cups (140 g) chopped kale

½ teaspoon ghee

½ teaspoon ground cumin

pinch of sea salt

Serves 2

First, prepare the quinoa. Put the broth in a saucepan and bring to a boil. Stir in the quinoa, cover, and cook over a low heat for 20 minutes or until tender and all the liquid has been absorbed.

Meanwhile, put 3 cups (700 ml) water in a large saucepan with a steamer basket and bring to the boil. Put the veggies for your dosha in the basket, cover, and steam for 15 minutes or until the vegetables are tender.

Transfer the vegetables to a bowl and add the ghee or oil and the spice and salt appropriate for your dosha. Add the quinoa, mix to combine, and serve. Any leftovers will keep for up to 5 days in an airtight container in the refrigerator.

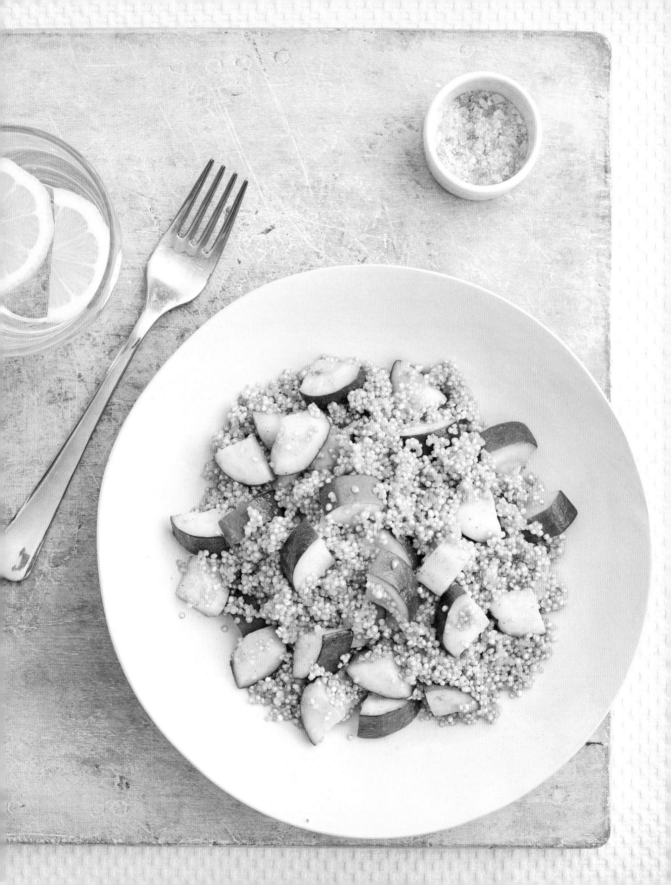

Breakfast Sweet Potato

Sweet potatoes nourish the liver, especially when eaten for breakfast (or before 10 a.m.–the prime time for nourishing the liver). If you want to get ahead, cook this dish the night before or increase the quantities so you make enough for the week ahead.

1 sweet potato

1 tablespoon sprouted almond butter

½ teaspoon ghee

½ teaspoon ground cinnamon

Serves 1

Preheat the oven to 450°F/230°C/Gas 8 and line a baking sheet with parchment (baking) paper.

Wash and clean your sweet potato and then use a fork to poke holes several times in the potato. Place the potato on the prepared baking sheet and bake in the oven for 40–45 minutes, until tender. To serve, transfer the potato to a plate, cut it in half, and top with the almond butter, ghee, and cinnamon.

If you cook in advance, the baked sweet potato will keep for up to 5 days in an airtight container in the refrigerator. To reheat, bake in an oven preheated to 350°F/180°C/Gas 4 for 10 minutes or cook in the microwave for 2 minutes.

Savory Oat Bowl

I love mixing up my meals and using breakfast foods for lunch or dinner. Oat bran is really versatile and can be used as a base for a quick nourishing meal. There are three different options for the veggies, oils, and spices, so choose the right one for your dosha.

FOR THE OAT BRAN

½ cup (50 g) gluten-free oat bran

2–3 cups (475–700 ml) water

FOR VATA

1 teaspoon ghee

1 teaspoon ground cumin

½ teaspoon ground fennel seeds

pinch of sea salt

pinch of ground black pepper

2 cups (260 g) chopped carrots

FOR PITTA

1 teaspoon coconut oil

1 teaspoon ground turmeric

½ teaspoon ground coriander

pinch of sea salt

2 cups (250 g) chopped zucchini (courgette)

FOR KAPHA

½ teaspoon ghee

1 teaspoon ground ginger

⅓ cup (5 g) chopped basil

pinch of sea salt

pinch of ground black pepper

3 cups (180 g) chopped spinach

Serves 2

Heat the ghee or oil, herbs and spices, and salt appropriate for your dosha in a saucepan over a medium heat. Add the water and oat bran and cook for 5 minutes (or according to instructions on the oat bran packet), stirring continuously, until the oats soften and thicken to a porridge consistency. Transfer the oat bran to a bowl and set aside.

Meanwhile, put 3 cups (700 ml) water in a large saucepan with a steamer basket and bring to the boil. Put the veggies for your dosha in the basket, cover, and steam for 15 minutes or until the vegetables are tender. Transfer the veggies to the oat bowl and enjoy. Any leftovers will keep for up to 5 days in an airtight container in the refrigerator.

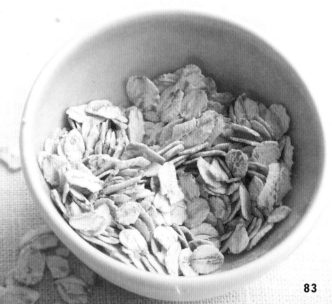

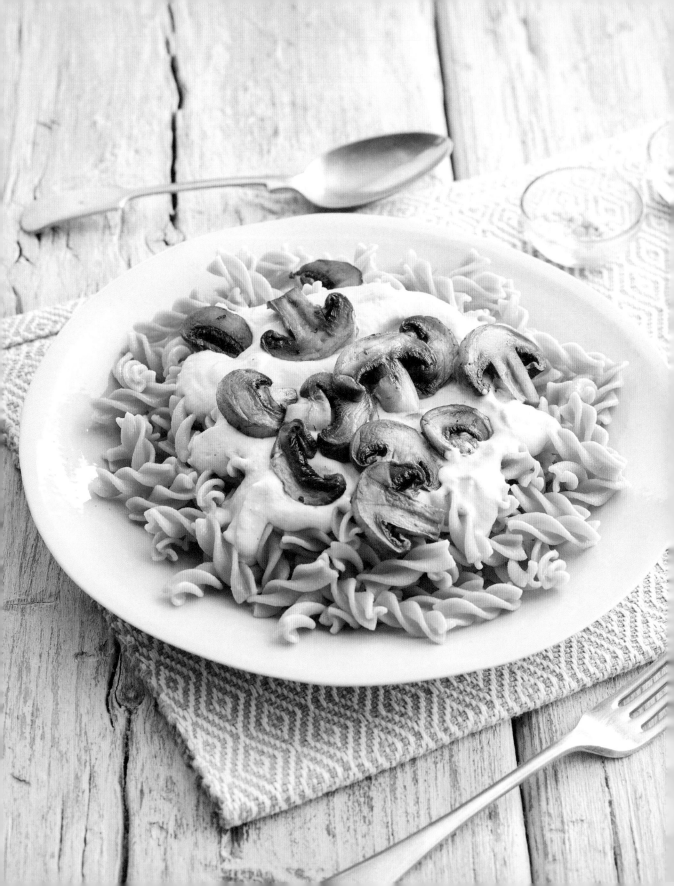

Chickpea Pasta with Cashew Cream Sauce

I love creamy sauces, the more sauce the better! Unfortunately, my body has never agreed with those heavy sauces, until I found the right swap. Cashews are dense in nutrients and they make the perfect Alfredo sauce or can be added to any sauce to make it creamy. Here, my Cashew Cream Sauce accompanies chickpea pasta and sautéed mushrooms, but I also love to pair it with zucchini (courgette) noodles. You can even use it as a vegan-friendly topping for nachos. Chickpea pasta is a healthier, more protein-rich alternative to wheat-based pasta.

8 oz (225 g) chickpea pasta

pinch of sea salt

1¼ teaspoons cold-pressed olive oil

2 cups (130 g) mushrooms, sliced

FOR THE CASHEW CREAM SAUCE

2 cups (240 g) cashews

1¼ cups (300 ml) water, plus extra to thin the sauce, if necessary

1 teaspoon sea salt

½ cup (25 g) nutritional yeast

3 pinches of ground coriander

1 teaspoon onion powder

1 teaspoon garlic powder

Serves 4

First make the cashew cream sauce. Place cashews in a bowl, add just enough water to cover the cashews, and let soak for 2 hours. Drain the cashews, and rinse thoroughly. Put the cashews in a food processor or blender, add all remaining sauce ingredients and blend until very, very smooth. If necessary, use a little water to thin out the sauce to your desired consistency.

Put 1 quart (1.1 liters) water in a large saucepan and bring to the boil. (Depending on the type of chickpea pasta you use, you may need to use more or less water.) Add the salt and ¼ teaspoon oil and cook according to the packet instructions.

While the pasta is cooking, heat the remaining oil in a sauté pan and add the mushrooms. Cook over a medium heat for 5–10 minutes, stirring occasionally, or until they begin to brown.

Drain the pasta well once cooked.

To serve, divide the pasta between bowls, spoon over the cream sauce, and add the mushrooms on top. Any leftover sauce will keep for up to 2 days in an airtight container in the refrigerator; and any leftover pasta will keep for up to 5 days in an airtight container in the refrigerator.

DESSERTS, SNACKS, AND COMFORT FOODS

Ayurveda is all about balance, for without moderation we either overindulge or restrict our eating to the point of discomfort. Neither of those options works for me, or my clients, which is why I make my own healthy treats to replace the junk-filled items that unfortunately I love. The recipes in this section, which are suitable for all the doshas, can be made for those times when you want to indulge—or even eaten daily!

Anandi's Ananda Raw Chocolate

Although the sweet taste is necessary in our daily diets, it should not be obtained from the consumption of white sugar, processed candies, or anything artificial. Luckily this chocolate is real, raw, and safe for everyday eats.

Raw cacao is a powerful medicinal superfood that has been used for centuries in many different cultures for its healing powers. It is rich in magnesium and iron, elevates mood and spirit, has forty times the antioxidants of blueberries (per serving), and contains more calcium than cow's milk. Raw cacao is also considered to be bliss-inducing due to its slow breakdown of the fatty acid neurotransmitter anandamide.

Ananda, which means "bliss" in Sanskrit, gives this raw chocolate its sacred name. I was given the spiritual name Anandi (also meaning "bliss") by an Ayurvedic astrological priest. He read my astrological chart and told me the sound my soul made when I was born was "anandi," and I kept this as a nickname.

This recipe is balancing to all three doshas, simply choose the sweetener option that best fits your dosha. Feel free to consume this raw chocolate in small doses (about 1½ oz/40 g daily) but be conscious of your consumption in the evenings if you are experiencing a Vata imbalance.

For an Herbal Aphrodisiac Raw Chocolate

Make the recipe as on the right, adding ½ teaspoon ashwagandha powder, ½ teaspoon pine pollen, and ½ teaspoon schizandra berry powder to the mixture with the cacao powder. The combination of these three adaptogens will increase blood flow to all the right parts, balance hormones, increase libido function, and give you an inner glow.

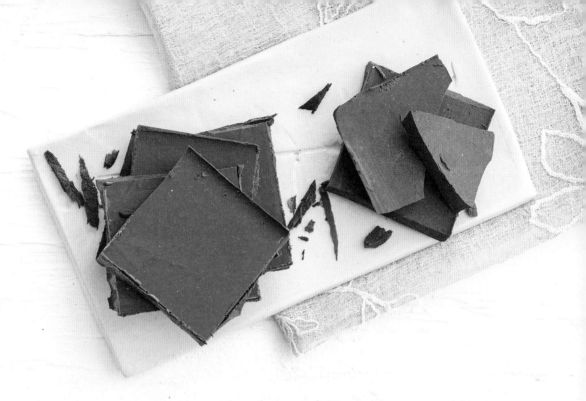

1 cup (220 g) raw cacao butter

1 cup (100 g) raw cacao powder

⅓ cup (75 ml) raw honey (for Vata); maple syrup–Grade B if possible (for Pitta); or liquid stevia drops or monk fruit sugar (for Kapha)

Makes 12 bars

Line an 8 x 8-inch (20 x 20-cm) baking pan with parchment (baking) paper. Alternatively, you can use a chocolate mold of your choice.

Melt the cacao butter in a double boiler (bain marie) over a very low heat (the lowest heat setting available). Add the cacao powder and mix until smooth. (I like to use a hand-held emulsion blender to achieve the smoothest chocolate.) Add the honey, maple syrup, stevia, or sugar and mix again.

Transfer the cacao mixture to the prepared baking pan or mold and place in the freezer for at least 30 minutes, until the chocolate is set. (Alternatively, you can chill it in the refrigerator overnight.)

Once the chocolate has hardened, turn it out of the pan and cut it into 12 squares, each about 2 x 2 inches (5 x 5 cm). The chocolate will keep for up to 2 weeks in an airtight container in the refrigerator or up to 1 month in the freezer.

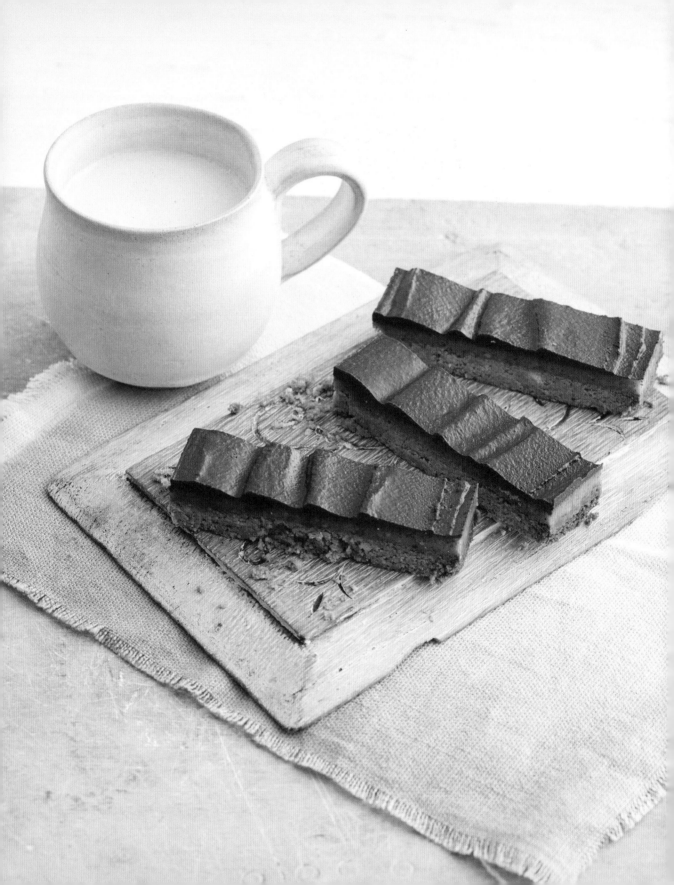

Grain-free Adaptogenic Chocolate Nougat Bar

Twix were my favorite candy when I was growing up. Being born on Halloween, I always received special treatment when I went trick-or-treating in my neighborhood and was able to sift through buckets to find my prized Twix. Fast forward to years later and my love for the caramel-and-chocolate covered cookie had yet to end. Of course, I needed to come up with a better way to enjoy my guilty pleasure without feeling completely ill. The result was this recipe, which includes two adaptogen stars: lucuma and maca.

FOR THE SHORTBREAD

2 cups (190 g) almond flour

2 tablespoons coconut flour

1 teaspoon vanilla bean powder

½ cup (120 ml) melted coconut oil

2 tablespoons lucuma powder

FOR THE CARAMEL

½ cup (125 g) almond butter, softened

⅓ cup (75 ml) melted coconut oil

⅓ cup (75 ml) maple syrup

¼ teaspoon sea salt

1 teaspoon vanilla bean powder

FOR THE CHOCOLATE

¼ cup (60 ml) melted coconut oil

¼ cup (25 g) cacao powder

2 tablespoons maple syrup

pinch of sea salt

2 tablespoons maca powder

Makes 16 bars

Preheat the oven to 350°F/180°C/Gas 4. Line an 8 x 8-inch (20 x 20-cm) baking pan with parchment (baking) paper.

To make the shortbread, put all the ingredients in a bowl and mix until well combined. Pour the mixture into the prepared pan and press it into the bottom of the pan. Bake in the oven for 11–13 minutes, or until the sides of the shortbread are lightly brown. Let cool.

Next, make the caramel. Put all the ingredients in a bowl and mix until completely smooth. Pour over cooled shortbread and chill in the refrigerator for 1–2 hours, until the caramel has hardened.

To prepare the chocolate mixture, put all the ingredients in a bowl and mix until smooth. (A whisk usually works best for mixing the chocolate.) Pour the chocolate over the caramel layer, and chill in the refrigerator for 1 hour, or until hardened.

To remove the candy from the pan, lift it up using the parchment paper and place it on a cutting board. Cut into 16 bars. The candy will keep for up to 1 week in an airtight container in the refrigerator or 1 month in the freezer.

Grain-free Blueberry Pop Tarts

I remember the days when my mom would send me off to school with a Pop-Tart in hand, and that was breakfast. I can't lie, I would still eat Pop-Tarts if I knew they were helping my health. Unfortunately, that isn't the case, so I've come up with a version of my own that is full of real food and will satisfy kids and adults alike. You can feel good about sending your little one off to school with one of these pop tarts as a snack or you can enjoy one yourself for breakfast, pairing it with a cup of tea.

FOR THE FILLING

2¾ cups (350 g) fresh or frozen blueberries

¼ cup (60 ml) maple syrup

2 tablespoons tapioca flour

FOR THE DOUGH

1¼ cups (120 g) almond flour

1 cup (125 g) tapioca flour

pinch of Himalayan pink salt

4 tablespoons cold-pressed coconut oil

1 egg

2 tablespoons maple syrup

Makes 4 pop tarts

First, prepare the filling. Put the blueberries and maple syrup in a saucepan and cook over a medium heat until the mixture starts to simmer, then turn down the heat and simmer, stirring all the time, until the blueberries begin to burst. Slowly add the tapioca flour and cook for a further 3 minutes or until the mixture begins to thicken. Remove from the heat and set aside to cool.

Preheat the oven to 350°F/180°C/Gas 4. Line a baking sheet with parchment (baking) paper.

To make the dough, put the flours and salt in a food processor or blender and pulse to combine. Add the oil and pulse until the mixture has a clumpy, sand-like consistency. Add the egg and maple syrup and process until a dough-like consistency forms.

On a work surface lined with parchment paper or a silicone mat, roll the dough into a 10 x 6-inch (25 x 15-cm) rectangle, about ¼ inch (5 mm) thick. Cut into 8 rectangles, each 5 x 3 inches (12.5 x 7.5 cm) in dimension.

Spread the filling over 4 of the rectangles, then cover each with one of the remaining rectangles. Use a fork to crimp the edges closed. Transfer the pop tarts to the prepared baking sheet and bake in the oven for 15–20 minutes, until golden brown. Let cool a little before eating and enjoy!

The pop tarts will keep for up to 1 week in an airtight container in the refrigerator or up to 1 month in the freezer. You can reheat in a toaster or bake in an oven preheated to 350°F/180°C/Gas 4 for 5–10 minutes.

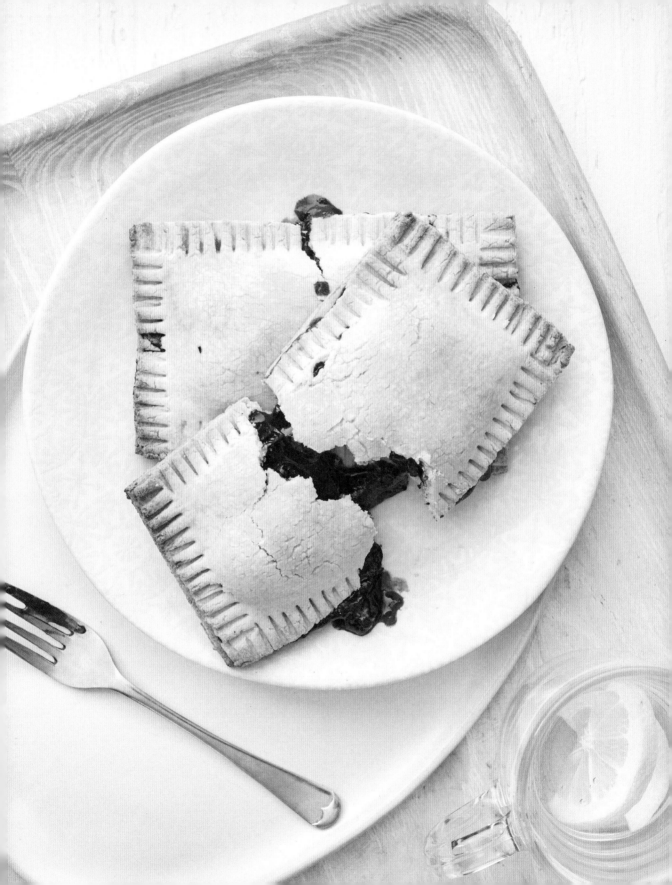

Lemon, Rose, and Poppy Seed Muffins

These muffins are a healthy version of a bakery classic, plus they have the added beauty benefit of rose water. Muffins are easy to bake ahead of time, making them a great snack to grab when you are on the go.

½ cup (45 g) coconut flour

½ teaspoon baking soda
(bicarbonate of soda)

1 tablespoon poppy seeds

1½ tablespoons grated lemon zest

juice of 1 large lemon

3 tablespoons rose water

⅓ cup (75 ml) melted coconut oil,
plus extra for greasing

4 drops of liquid stevia

½ cup (120 ml) unsweetened
almond milk

3 eggs

Makes 12 muffins

Preheat the oven to 325°F/160°C/Gas 3. Make sure all your ingredients are at room temperature before you start making the batter. Grease a 12-cup nonstick muffin pan with coconut oil.

In a large bowl, combine the flour, baking soda (bicarbonate of soda), poppy seeds, and lemon zest. In a separate large bowl, combine the lemon juice, rose water, oil, stevia, milk, and eggs. Pour the wet ingredients into the dry ingredients and mix well.

Spoon the batter into the cups of the prepared muffin pan. Bake in the oven for 20–25 minutes, until golden brown and a skewer inserted into the center comes out clean.

Remove from oven and let cool in the pan. The muffins will keep for up to 1 week in an airtight container in the refrigerator or up to 1 month in the freezer.

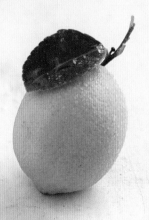

Lavender and Coconut Cookies

I often crave cookies because I'm human, just like everyone else. Whether it's cookies and milk or cookies and tea, they are all delicious to me. Eat my Lavender and Coconut Cookies as a snack with a digestive tea or adaptogenic tonic (see pages 98–109). You can eat two cookies per serving.

1 very ripe banana (the skin should be almost all brown), peeled

2 drops of food-grade lavender essential oil (I use Young Living's Lavender Vitality essential oil, see page 156)

¼ teaspoon pure vanilla extract or powder

⅔ cup (45 g) unsweetened shredded coconut

Makes 8 cookies

Preheat the oven to 350°F/180°C/Gas 4. Line a baking sheet with parchment (baking) paper.

Put the banana, lavender oil, and vanilla in a bowl and mash them together until smooth. Stir in the coconut until the mixture looks like dry mashed potatoes.

Using a tablespoon, scoop out 2 tablespoonfuls of the cookie dough and roll them into a ball. Place the ball on the prepared baking sheet and repeat until you have used up all the cookie dough. Using a fork, press down the cookies until they are about ½ inch (1 cm) thick. Bake in the oven for 11 minutes or until golden brown.

Remove from the oven and let cool on a wire rack. The cookies will keep for up to 5 days in an airtight container in the refrigerator.

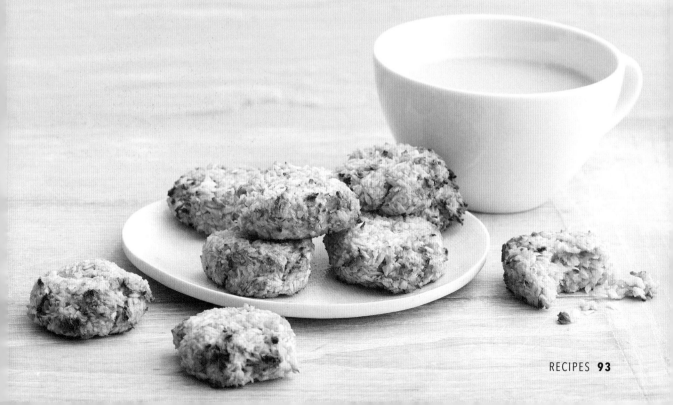

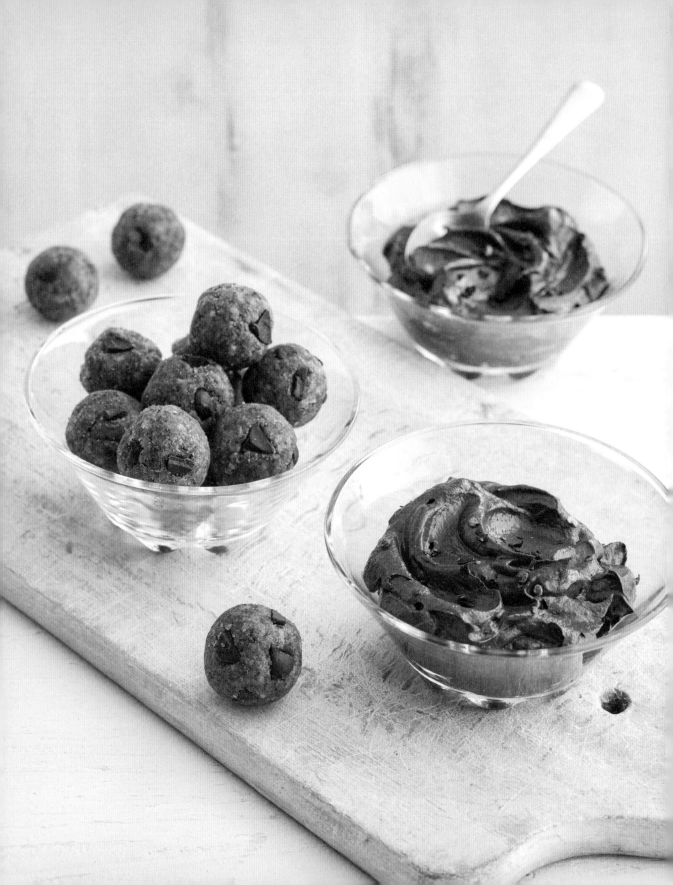

Raw Cookie Dough Bites

There will be no more feeling sick and guilty for eating raw cookie dough! This cookie dough is actually packed with protein and makes a delicious snack or topping for yogurt bowls.

1 x 14-oz (400-g) can of chickpeas, drained and rinsed

2 teaspoons pure vanilla extract

¼ cup plus 1 tablespoon (175 g) flax meal (ground flax seeds)

¼ teaspoon Himalayan pink salt

½ cup (120 ml) maple syrup or other liquid sweetener

⅛ teaspoon baking soda (bicarbonate of soda)

½ cup (75 g) stevia-sweetened chocolate chips

Makes about 16 dough bites

Combine all the ingredients in a food processor or blender and blend for about 15 seconds or until the mixture is well combined, stopping once to scrape down the sides.

Roll the mixture into little balls and place in an airtight container. The dough bites will keep for up to 5 days in an airtight container in the refrigerator or up to 1 month in the freezer.

Sexy Mexican Chocolate and Avocado Mousse

This dessert is for those nights when you just need to indulge in something with a smooth kick.

¼ teaspoon chipotle chili powder

1 teaspoon pine pollen powder

2 ripe avocados, peeled and stoned

½ cup (50 g) raw cacao powder

½ cup (120 ml) full-fat coconut milk

⅓ cup (75 ml) maple syrup

1 teaspoon ground cinnamon

2 teaspoons pure vanilla extract

Serves 2–3

Combine all the ingredients in a food processor or blender and blend until completely smooth. Taste and adjust the seasoning if necessary. Spoon the mixture into 2 or 3 small serving dishes and chill in the refrigerator until set. The mousse will keep for up to 5 days in the refrigerator.

Grain-free Orange Zest Pancakes

I'm a pancake lover and these zesty pancakes hit the right spot. They are the most guilt-free indulgence you'll ever have for breakfast. The orange is especially balancing to Kapha (although suitable for all doshas) and invigorating when eaten in the morning. If you prefer, you can replace the orange with another flavor.

1 cup (95 g) almond flour

¾ cup (95 g) tapioca flour

1 tablespoon baking powder

¼ teaspoon sea salt

⅓ cup (75 ml) unsweetened almond milk

2 teaspoons apple cider vinegar

1 tablespoon maple syrup

1 tablespoon coconut oil, plus extra for greasing

1 teaspoon pure vanilla extract

2 drops of food-grade sweet orange essential oil (I use Young Living's Sweet Orange Vitality essential oil, see page 156)

1 teaspoon grated orange zest (optional)

4 teaspoons ghee, for topping

Serves 2

First, make the batter. Combine all the ingredients except the orange zest and ghee in a food processor or blender and blend for a few seconds, then scrape down the sides and blend for a few seconds longer. (Blending helps to make these egg-free pancakes fluffier.) Transfer the batter to a bowl and fold in the orange zest, if using.

Heat a nonstick or cast-iron skillet (frying pan) over a medium heat. Dip a scrunched-up piece of kitchen paper into the oil and carefully use this to grease the hot skillet. Drop one quarter of the batter into the skillet and cook for 3–5 minutes, until you see little bubbles forming on the surface of the pancake and the underside is golden brown. Flip the pancake and cook for a further 3–5 minutes. Keep the patties warm while you cook the remaining batter, greasing the pan with a little more oil if necessary. To serve, divide the pancakes between 2 plates and top each pancake with 1 teaspoon of ghee. Any leftover pancakes will keep for up to 2 days in an airtight container in the refrigerator.

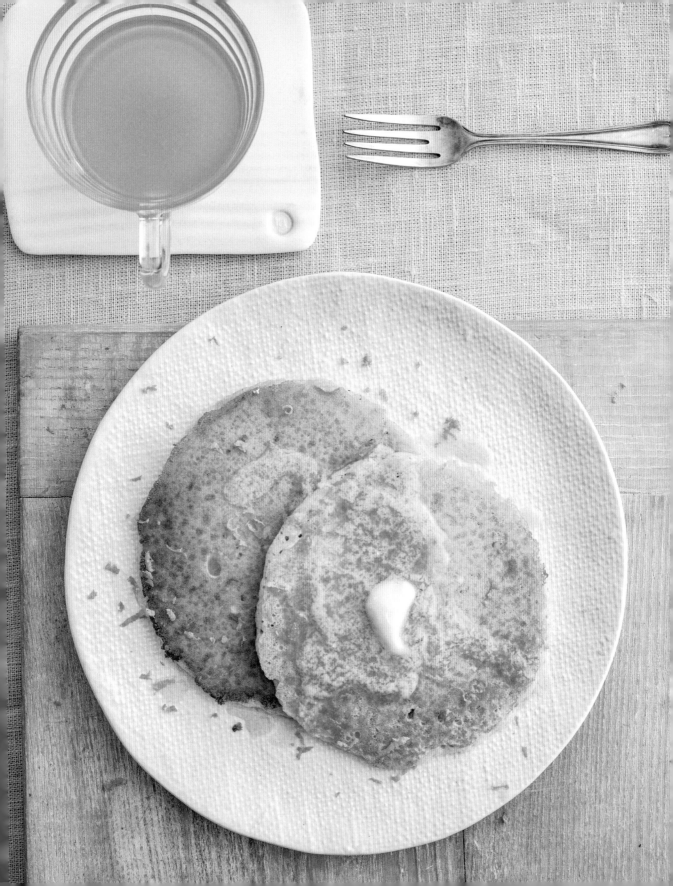

INGEST: TREAT YOUR INSIDES RIGHT WITH TEA

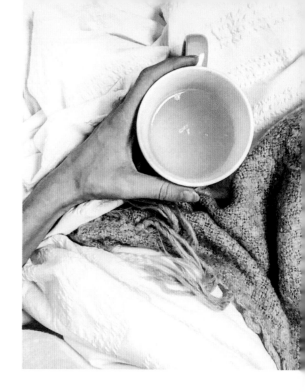

By now you should understand that what we put in (and on) our bodies has a direct relationship to our health and well-being. We can use plant medicine to heal our bodies and evoke feelings of self-love.

Gentle Detox Tea

This age-old Ayurvedic recipe boosts detoxification. In particular, it works wonders if you have been indulging a little too much while on vacation or are battling a post-pizza party belly. The fennel reduces gas and bloating, the cumin helps to balance blood sugar, the coriander acts as a calming agent, and the manjistha is an anti-inflammatory and clears the lymphatic system. Drink this tea daily if you're struggling regularly with constant gas, bloating, indigestion, acid reflux, or sluggish digestion. If you suffer from any of these symptoms, there's no need to buy fancy pills or supplements for a rescue detox, just reach for your spice rack and brew up a pot of this tea! Daily use of this tea will not only promote a gentle full body detox but also facilitate fat burning, aid in the digestion of proteins, and balance all three doshas.

4–5 cups (950 ml–1.2 liters) water

½ **teaspoon cumin seeds**

½ **teaspoon coriander seeds**

½ **teaspoon fennel seeds**

½ **teaspoon manjistha powder**

Serves 4

Put the water in a saucepan and bring to the boil. Add the remaining ingredients, cover, and let boil for 5 minutes. Using a strainer or cheesecloth (muslin), strain the tea and pour into a thermos.

Take small sips of the tea throughout the day or drink 1 cup (250 ml) of the tea before or after meals.

Weight-loss Tea

It's important to know there is no quick or easy way to lose weight—as with everything in life, it takes time and consistency. However, there are plenty of things you can do on a daily basis to encourage weight loss and weight maintenance. This recipe is best for people with excess Kapha or out of balance Kapha; other doshas can also use the tea for weight loss, but only in moderation. Basil is not usually found in common weight-loss teas but often weight gain can be due to over-toxicity in the body, especially the liver. Basil promotes detoxification of the liver, functions as an adaptogen in the body, and is an anti-inflammatory. Green tea is rich in antioxidants, stabilizes blood sugar levels, and is rich in EGCG (epigallocatechin gallate—a polyphenol found in tea), which helps to combat obesity. Combined with lemon, ginger, and raw honey, this metabolism-boosting beverage can be enjoyed daily.

4–5 cups (950 ml–1.2 liters) water

1 teaspoon chopped fresh basil or ½–1 teaspoon dried basil

2 teaspoons green tea leaves

1-inch (2.5-cm) piece of fresh ginger, peeled and chopped

juice of 1 lemon

½ teaspoon raw honey

Serves 4

Put the water in a saucepan and bring to the boil. Add all the remaining ingredients except the honey, cover, and let boil for 5 minutes. Using a strainer or cheesecloth (muslin), strain the tea and pour into a thermos.

Once the tea has cooled to a warm temperature (see below), add the raw honey. Drink the tea throughout the day.

Raw Honey

When using raw honey, never add the honey to boiling or very hot water. Heat changes the medicinal properties of raw honey, making it turn to excess toxins in the body instead of healing the body. Only add the honey to teas, or other dishes, when they have cooled to a warm temperature.

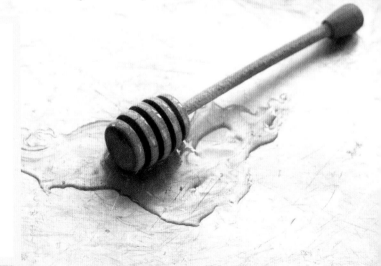

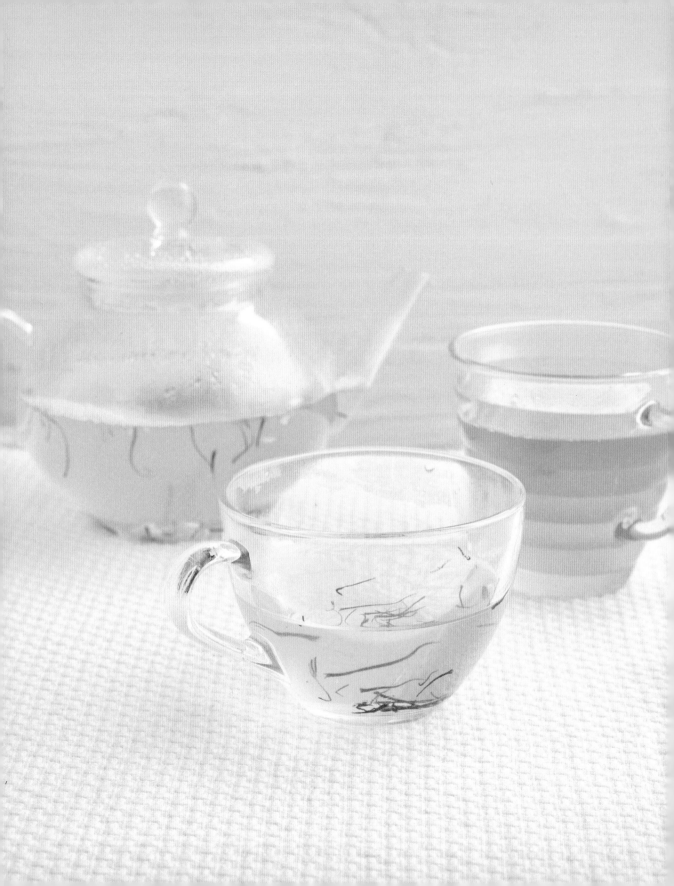

Digestive Rose Tea

Drinking herbal tea is like taking a supplement. It's an easy way to take in nature's medicine and can become a soothing act of kindness. This recipe is best for people with a high Pitta constitution or a Pitta imbalance. The cardamom enhances digestion while also calming indigestion and heartburn. The fennel is a potent digestive aid and works wonders in combination with fresh ginger, which is an all-round healer. When ginger is taken before meals it aids in the absorption of nutrients. The rose is cooling and calming in nature, which makes it the perfect partner to balance out these other heating herbs. Rose is rich in vitamin C and revered as a beauty herb.

4–5 cups (950 ml–1.2 liters) water

½ teaspoon cardamom pods

½ teaspoon fennel seeds

¼-inch (5-mm) piece of fresh ginger, peeled and chopped

½ teaspoon dried rose buds

Put the water in a saucepan and bring to the boil. Add all the remaining ingredients, cover, and let boil for 5 minutes. Using a strainer or cheesecloth (muslin), strain the tea and pour into a thermos.

Enjoy the tea with snacks or drink it throughout the day for a calming digestive tonic.

Serves 4

Saffron and Lemon Elixir

Saffron is widely used in Ayurvedic medicine for its ability to beautify the skin, boost moods, decrease feelings of depression, and combat PMS and infertility in both men and women. This elixir is beneficial to all three doshas.

½-inch (1-cm) piece of fresh ginger, peeled and grated

½ teaspoon saffron threads

juice of 1 lemon

2 tablespoons monk fruit sugar

4–5 cups (950 ml–1.2 liters) water

Put the ginger, saffron, lemon juice, and monk fruit sugar in a small saucepan over a low heat, then add the water and let the liquid come to the boil. Remove from the heat, cover, and let stand for 20 minutes.

There's no need to strain this tea. Pour the liquid into a thermos and enjoy the tea hot or at room temperature. I also like to freeze the tea in ice-cube trays and add the ice cubes to room-temperature water– the ice cubes make the water a beautiful color.

Serves 4

Quiet Mind Tea

If you ever feel overwhelmed and stressed out, it's a signal to your body to carve out some time for self-love. When we overload ourselves with stress and anxiety, our bodies can break down, and no matter how much good we think we are doing, we need to take time to heal. Taking a break from your everyday tasks to relax and quiet the mind is an important part of the self-healing process. If you don't nourish yourself, you won't be able to nourish anyone else. This recipe is perfect to calm Vata and Pitta. Pair the tea with the Relaxing Chamomile Bath (see page 138). The tea's combination of four herbs works on the nervous system to calm feelings of being on edge and will instantly send you into a blissful state of relaxation. Brahmi is one of the ancient herbs in Ayurvedic medicine. It is considered a nervine tonic due to its ability to intensely calm the nervous system and boost memory. Chamomile and lavender are anti-inflammatory and they bring a sense of peace and clarity to the body and mind. (You'll find these two herbs in many over-the-counter sleep teas.) Valerian is a powerful root that is actually considered nature's Valium. Valerian root works wonders for people suffering from anxiety, insomnia, chronic stress, and severe muscle cramps (it's great for menstrual pains).

1 tablespoon dried brahmi leaf

1 tablespoon dried lavender flowers

1 tablespoon dried chamomile flowers

½ tablespoon dried valerian root

2 cups (475 ml) boiled water

raw honey, to taste

Serves 2

Put the herbs and boiled water in a bowl and let the mixture steep for 5 minutes. (If you oversteep the herbs, this tea will become very bitter and won't be as pleasant to drink.) Using a strainer or cheesecloth (muslin), strain the tea and pour into a thermos.

Once the tea has cooled to a warm temperature (see page 99), add the raw honey and enjoy!

Beauty Ambrosia Tea

This is one of my favorite teas to incorporate into my self-love rituals. I usually it pair with a face mask and raw chocolate. The word *ambrosia* means "immortality" in Greek. If you want clear, radiant, glowing skin, it must come from within—what we put on our skin is just an extra bonus. Hibiscus, rose, and calendula all pacify Pitta and also help to remove excess heat from the blood, heal the heart, and tonify the skin for all three doshas. I suggest investing in a bulk quantity of these dried flowers (see page 156) so you always have the ingredients to hand to make this tea.

3 tablespoons dried hibiscus flowers

2 tablespoons dried calendula flowers

2 tablespoons dried red or pink rose petals

2 cups (475 ml) boiled water

raw honey, to taste

Serves 2

Put the herbs and boiled water in a bowl and let the mixture steep for 1 hour or until the liquid is a vibrant red color. Using a strainer or cheesecloth (muslin), strain the tea and pour into a thermos.

Once the tea has cooled to a warm temperature (see page 99), add the raw honey. Enjoy the tea warm or at room temperature.

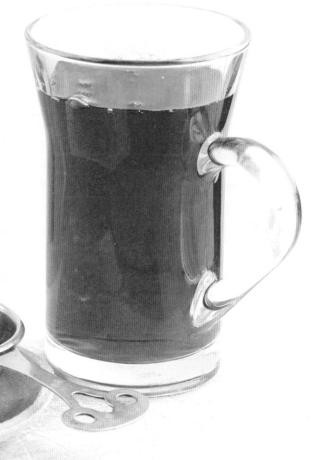

Vitali-Tea

Oftentimes when we don't pay attention to ourselves we become unconscious of what we are putting in our bodies, which can lead to sluggishness and stagnation of lymph tissues. It's important to show your body respect and honor the powerful things it does for you on a daily basis. Incorporating rituals and taking in plant medicine is a wonderful way to bring awareness back to the self. Anything we do for ourselves that enhances joy, love, and happiness is a form of self-love. Vitali-Tea is a special way not only to balance Kapha but also to help stimulate the body and mind for all three doshas. It is also a great tea to enjoy when you need to detox, paired with a self-massage (see page 132) and sweet orange and ginger essential oils (see page 130). The liver and kidneys play an important role in keeping our bodies clean. When we support these two organs, we are aiding the body in the process of detoxification. Dandelion root is one of the best remedies for supporting the liver. It is also revered as a diuretic and can help reduce water retention. Licorice root supports the digestive system and helps push extra toxins out of our organs. Cinnamon and cardamom are warming, which helps to balance the cool dampness of Kapha. Orange peel is slightly heating and super rich in vitamin C.

1 tablespoon licorice root

1 tablespoon dandelion root

½ tablespoon dried orange peel

½ teaspoon cardamom seeds

¼ teaspoon cinnamon chips

2 cups (475 ml) boiled water

raw honey, to taste

Serves 2

Put the herbs and boiled water in a bowl and let the mixture steep for 20 minutes. (Since we are working with roots, its best to let the tea steep for longer than we do when making teas with leaves or flowers.) Using a strainer or cheesecloth (muslin), strain the tea and pour into a thermos.

Once the tea has cooled to a warm temperature (see page 99), add the raw honey and enjoy!

TONICS:
HERBAL LIFESTYLE
ENHANCEMENTS

As well as teas, you can also drink Ayurvedic tonics for health and well-being. The tonic recipes I recommend in this chapter all harness the healing properties of adaptogens.

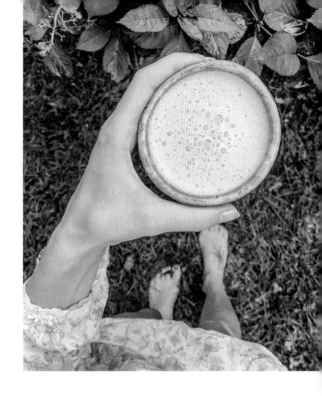

Adaptogenic Sleep Milk

I came up with this tonic because I was experiencing horrible bouts of insomnia. Pair the tonic with a warm bath or sleep ritual to enhance the dreamy vibes. The ghee is grounding and nourishing, which is perfect right before sleep. This sleep milk is suitable for all three doshas, though Kapha rarely needs help sleeping.

1 teaspoon ghee

½ tablespoon ashwagandha powder

½ tablespoon mucuna pruriens powder

½ teaspoon astragalus powder

1½ cups (350 ml) warm almond milk (or other nut milk)

1 teaspoon raw honey

Serves 1

Heat the ghee in a saucepan over a low heat for 1 minute, then add the herbs and simmer for 30 seconds. Add the milk and stir. (If you have a hand-held milk frother or whisk, you may use it to froth the milk.) Remove from the heat.

Once the liquid has cooled to a warm temperature (see page 99), add the honey.

Adaptogenic Beauty Milk

Use this powerful beauty milk daily to build your radiance from within and achieve glowing clear skin and radiant hair. It is suitable for all three doshas.

1½ cups (350 ml) water

½ cup (120 ml) almond milk

1 tablespoon pearl powder

1 tablespoon amalaki powder

½ tablespoon schizandra berry

1 teaspoon raw honey

Serves 1

Put the water and almond milk in a small saucepan and cook over a low heat for 3 minutes or until it comes to a low boil.

Transfer the mixture to a food processor or blender, add all the remaining ingredients except the honey, and blend on high until the milk gets frothy.

Once the liquid has cooled to a warm temperature (see page 99), add the honey. Drink out of your favorite mug.

Moringa Morning Matcha Tonic

I love green tea and my all-time favorite is matcha. If you've never tried matcha, it's one of the most decadent and velvety smooth teas you'll ever taste. Matcha is rich in EGCG (see page 99), which is crucial for antiaging. Probably you won't find moringa and matcha combined at your local tea or coffee shop, but this is an easy pick-me-up you can make at home. You don't need professional matcha tea equipment, just a small bowl and a whisk.

½ cup (120 ml) almond milk

1 teaspoon matcha green tea powder

¼ cup (60 ml) hot water

½ teaspoon moringa powder

½ teaspoon mucuna pruriens powder

raw honey or stevia, to taste

Serves 1

Heat the almond milk in a small saucepan over a medium-low heat for 3 minutes or until the milk slightly bubbles.

Meanwhile, put the matcha in a small bowl and add the hot water. Whisk until the matcha has completely dissolved and become smooth.

Transfer the almond milk to a food processor or blender, add the moringa and mucuna pruriens, and blend until smooth. Pour into a mug, top with the matcha, and stir together. Once the liquid has cooled to a warm temperature (see page 99), add the honey or stevia.

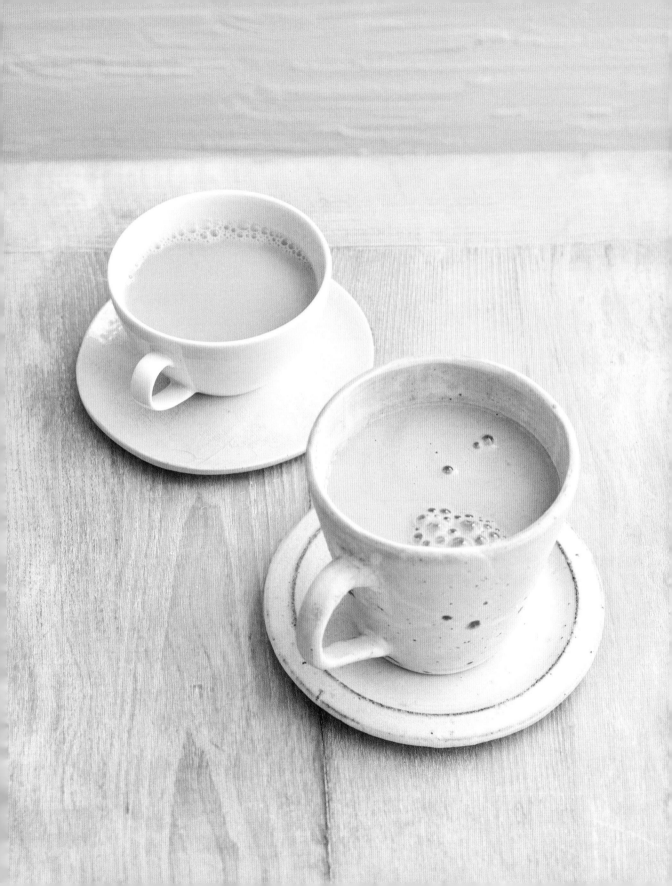

Deep Chocolate Elixir

Instead of coffee, I turn to adaptogens and raw cacao to satisfy my energy needs. This tonic is sure to send your blood circulating to all the right places. Drink this with a partner or by yourself and let the creative juices flow.

1 cup (250 ml) water

¼ cup (60 ml) almond milk

½ teaspoon ground cinnamon

½ teaspoon ground cardamom

1 teaspoon pure vanilla extract or powder

2 teaspoons pine pollen powder

1 teaspoon he shou wu powder

¼ cup (25 g) raw cacao powder

1 tablespoon coconut oil

raw honey, to taste

Serves 1

Put the water and almond milk in a small saucepan and cook over a low heat for 3 minutes or until it comes to a low boil. Add all the remaining ingredients except the raw honey.

Transfer the mixture to a food processor or blender and blend for 1–2 minutes, until smooth and frothy.

Once the liquid has cooled to a warm temperature (see page 99), pour into a mug and add the raw honey.

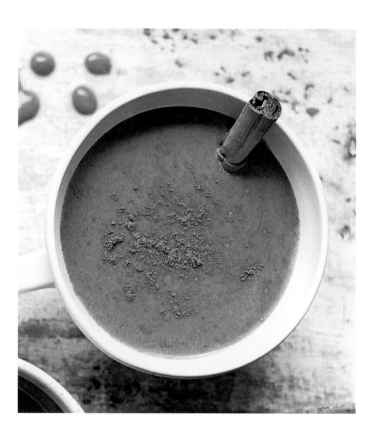

Ashwagandha Chai Latte

Chai tea was one of the first teas I found myself gravitating toward at the start of my journey with Ayurvedic medicine. The aromas and velvety warmth of a cup of chai feels like a big hug to the soul. I often start my day with this upgraded version of a traditional chai latte.

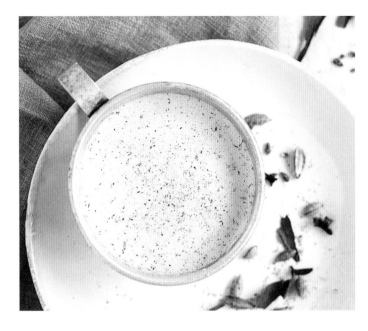

3 cups (700 ml) unsweetened almond milk

½-inch (1-cm) piece of fresh ginger, peeled

1 tablespoon rooibos tea

2 star anise

2 cardamom pods

½ teaspoon whole cloves

1 cinnamon stick or ½ teaspoon cinnamon chips

1 teaspoon ashwagandha powder

½ teaspoon rhodiola powder

1 teaspoon sweetener of your choice, such as raw honey, maple syrup, or monk fruit sugar

Serves 2–3

Put the almond milk, ginger, rooibos tea, star anise, cardamom, cloves, and cinnamon in a small saucepan, cover, and bring the mixture to the boil. Remove from the heat and let stand, still covered, for 3–5 minutes, until the milk has darkened in color and smells aromatic.

Using a strainer or cheesecloth (muslin), strain the tea into a bowl and discard the herbs. Add the ashwagandha and rhodiola and mix well. Pour your chai into your favorite mug and add your sweetener of choice. If using raw honey, let the chai cool to a warm temperature before adding the honey (see page 99). Enjoy this tonic warm.

7-Day Meal Plans for Vata, Pitta, and Kapha

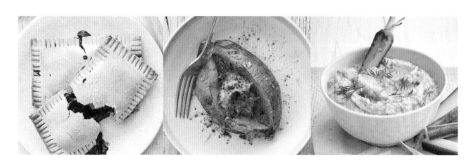

DAY 1

Morning beverage: Drink 1½–3¾ cups (350–900 ml) Warm Water with Fresh Lemon Juice with grated ginger (see page 52) first thing in the morning

Breakfast: Vata Breakfast Bowl (see page 63) and Moringa Morning Matcha Tonic (see page 106)

Snack: Grain-free Blueberry Pop Tart (see page 90) and Gentle Detox Tea (see page 98)

Lunch: Chickpea Pasta with Cashew Cream Sauce (see page 85)

Dinner: Cauliflower Tikka Masala (see page 64)

Dessert: Raw Cookie Dough Bite (see page 95)

Night cap: Adaptogenic Sleep Milk (see page 105)

DAY 2

Morning beverage: Drink 1½–3¾ cups (350–900 ml) Warm Water with Fresh Lemon Juice with grated ginger (see page 52) first thing in the morning

Breakfast: Breakfast Sweet Potato (see page 82)

Snack: Chris's Travel Shake (see page 67) and Gentle Detox Tea (see page 98)

Lunch: Lemon and Thyme Potatoes with Mixed Salad Greens (see page 76) and 1 cup (250 ml) low-sodium vegetable or bone broth

Dinner: Quinoa Bowl with Veggies (see page 80)

Dessert: Sexy Mexican Chocolate and Avocado Mousse (see page 95)

Night cap: Adaptogenic Sleep Milk (see page 105)

DAY 3

Morning beverage: Drink 1½–3¾ cups (350–900 ml) Warm Water with Fresh Lemon Juice with grated ginger (see page 52) first thing in the morning

Breakfast: Ashwaghanda Chai Latte (see page 109) and 1 banana

Snack: Chris's Travel Shake (see page 67)

Lunch: Spiced Sweet Potato Fries (see page 67) with store-bought hummus or Cucumber and Dill Hummus (see page 72) and Gentle Detox Tea (see page 98)

Dinner: Savory Oat Bowl (see page 83)

Dessert: Anandi's Ananda Raw Chocolate (see page 86)

Night cap: Adaptogenic Sleep Milk (see page 105)

I've created a 7-day meal plan for each dosha . You don't have to follow your dosha-specific meal plan exactly, it is simply here to help guide you with suggestions and recommendations. You may find that recipes that have been recommended for other doshas are in your meal plan; this is because, when paired properly, any food can be balancing to each dosha.

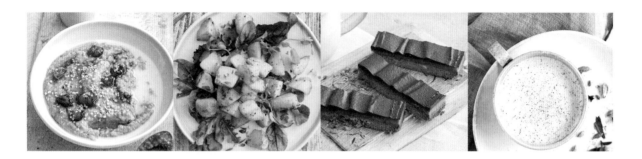

DAY 4

Morning beverage: Drink 1½–3¾ cups (350–900 ml) Warm Water with Fresh Lemon Juice with grated ginger (see page 52) first thing in the morning

Breakfast: Vata Breakfast Bowl (see page 63) and Moringa Morning Matcha Tonic (see page 106)

Snack: Grain-free Blueberry Pop Tart (see page 90) and Gentle Detox Tea (see page 98)

Lunch: Chickpea Pasta with Cashew Cream Sauce (see page 85)

Dinner: Cauliflower Tikka Masala (see page 64)

Dessert: Raw Cookie Dough Bite (see page 95)

Night cap: Adaptogenic Sleep Milk (see page 105)

DAY 5

Morning beverage: Drink 1½–3¾ cups (350–900 ml) Warm Water with Fresh Lemon Juice with grated ginger (see page 52) first thing in the morning

Breakfast: Chris's Travel Shake (see page 67) and Vata Breakfast Bowl (see page 63)

Snack: Spiced Sweet Potato Fries (see page 67) and Gentle Detox Tea (see page 98)

Lunch: Lemon and Thyme Potatoes with Mixed Salad Greens (see page 76) and 1 cup (250 ml) low-sodium vegetable or bone broth

Dinner: Quinoa Bowl with Veggies (see page 80)

Dessert: Sexy Mexican Chocolate and Avocado Mousse (see page 95)

Night cap: Adaptogenic Sleep Milk (see page 105)

DAY 6

Morning beverage: Drink 1½–3¾ cups (350–900 ml) Warm Water with Fresh Lemon Juice with grated ginger (see page 52) first thing in the morning

Breakfast: Ashwaghanda Chai Latte (see page 109) and 1 banana

Snack: Lala's Detox Smoothie (see page 79)

Lunch: Cauliflower Tikka Masala (see page 64) and Gentle Detox Tea (see page 98)

Dinner: Breakfast Sweet Potato (see page 82) with Beautifying Guacamole (see page 79)

Dessert: Grain-free Adaptogenic Chocolate Nougat Bar (see page 89)

Night cap: Adaptogenic Sleep Milk (see page 105)

DAY 7

Morning beverage: Drink 1½–3¾ cups (350–900 ml) Warm Water with Fresh Lemon Juice with grated ginger (see page 52) first thing in the morning

Breakfast: Ashwaghanda Chai Latte (see page 109) and 1 banana

Snack: Chris's Travel Shake (see page 67)

Lunch: Spiced Sweet Potato Fries (see page 67) with store-bought hummus or Cucumber and Dill Hummus (see page 72) and Gentle Detox Tea (see page 98)

Dinner: Savory Oat Bowl (see page 83)

Dessert: Grain-free Adaptogenic Chocolate Nougat Bar (see page 89)

Night cap: Adaptogenic Sleep Milk (see page 105)

7-DAY MEAL PLAN FOR PITTA

DAY 1

Morning beverage: Drink 1½–3¾ cups (350–900 ml) Warm Water with Fresh Lemon Juice (see page 52) first thing in the morning

Breakfast: Celery Juice Elixir (see page 53) and Beauty Breakfast Pudding (see page 68)

Snack: Logan's Tropical Smoothie (see page 72)

Lunch: Turmeric Patty Sandwich with Mint and Cilantro Dressing (see page 71)

Snack: Cucumber and Dill Hummus (see page 72) with celery sticks and Digestive Rose Tea (see page 101)

Dinner: Quinoa Bowl with Veggies (see page 80)

Dessert: Grain-free Adaptogenic Chocolate Nougat Bar (see page 89)

Night cap: Adaptogenic Beauty Milk (see page 106)

DAY 2

Morning beverage: Drink 1½–3¾ cups (350–900 ml) Warm Water with Fresh Lemon Juice (see page 52) first thing in the morning

Breakfast: Celery Juice Elixir (see page 53) and Grain-free Orange Zest Pancakes (see page 96)

Snack: Grain-free Blueberry Pop Tart (see page 90)

Lunch: Chickpea Pasta with Cashew Cream Sauce (see page 85)

Snack: Lavender and Coconut Cookie (see page 93) and Digestive Rose Tea (see page 101)

Dinner: Savory Oat Bowl (see page 83)

Dessert: Anandi's Ananda Raw Chocolate (see page 86)

Night cap: Adaptogenic Beauty Milk (see page 106)

DAY 3

Morning beverage: Drink 1½–3¾ cups (350–900 ml) Warm Water with Fresh Lemon Juice (see page 52) first thing in the morning

Breakfast: Celery Juice Elixir (see page 53) and warm oat bran made with coconut milk

Snack: Deep Chocolate Elixir (see page 108) and Lemon, Rose, and Poppy Seed Muffin (see page 92)

Lunch: Lemon and Thyme Potatoes with Mixed Salad Greens (see page 76) and Digestive Rose Tea (see page 101)

Snack: Logan's Tropical Smoothie (see page 72)

Dinner: Turmeric Patty Sandwich (see page 71), replacing the Mint and Cilantro Dressing with Cucumber and Dill Hummus (see page 72)

Dessert: Raw Cookie Dough Bite (see page 95)

Night cap: Adaptogenic Beauty Milk (see page 106)

7-DAY MEAL PLAN FOR KAPHA

DAY 1

Morning beverage: Drink 1½–3¾ cups (350–900 ml) Warm Water with Fresh Lemon Juice with raw honey (see page 52) first thing in the morning

Breakfast: Lala's Detox Smoothie (see page 79)

Lunch: Spring Herbed Frittata (see page 75) and Weight-loss Tea (see page 99)

Dinner: Grain-free Orange Zest Pancakes (see page 96)

Dessert: Anandi's Ananda Raw Chocolate (see page 86)

Night cap: Saffron and Lemon Elixir (see page 101)

DAY 2

Morning beverage: Drink 1½–3¾ cups (350–900 ml) Warm Water with Fresh Lemon Juice with raw honey (see page 52) first thing in the morning

Breakfast: Lala's Detox Smoothie (see page 79)

Lunch: Lemon and Thyme Potatoes with Mixed Salad Greens (see page 76) and Weight-loss Tea (see page 99)

Dinner: Cooked quinoa and steamed veggies in a low-sodium broth

Dessert: Grain-free Adaptogenic Chocolate Nougat Bar (see page 89)

Night cap: Saffron and Lemon Elixir (see page 101)

DAY 3

Morning beverage: Drink 1½–3¾ cups (350–900 ml) Warm Water with Fresh Lemon Juice with raw honey (see page 52) first thing in the morning

Breakfast: Lala's Detox Smoothie (see page 79)

Lunch: Turmeric Patty Sandwich with Mint and Cilantro Dressing (see page 71) with mixed salad greens dressed with lemon juice and Weight-loss Tea (see page 99)

Dinner: Savory Oat Bowl (see page 83)

Dessert: Raw Cookie Dough Bite (see page 95)

Night cap: Saffron and Lemon Elixir (see page 101)

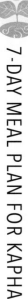

DAY 4

Morning beverage: Drink 1½–3¾ cups (350–900 ml) Warm Water with Fresh Lemon Juice (see page 52) first thing in the morning
Breakfast: Celery Juice Elixir (see page 53) and Beauty Breakfast Pudding (see page 68)
Snack: Beautifying Guacamole (see page 79) with cucumber slices
Lunch: Savory Oat Bowl (see page 83)
Snack: Lavender and Coconut Cookie (see page 93) and Digestive Rose Tea (see page 101)
Dinner: Chickpea Pasta with Cashew Cream Sauce (see page 85)
Dessert: Grain-free Adaptogenic Chocolate Nougat Bar (see page 89)
Night cap: Adaptogenic Beauty Milk (see page 106)

DAY 5

Morning beverage: Drink 1½–3¾ cups (350–900 ml) Warm Water with Fresh Lemon Juice (see page 52) first thing in the morning
Breakfast: Celery Juice Elixir (see page 53) and Grain-free Orange Zest Pancakes (see page 96)
Snack: Deep Chocolate Elixir (see page 108) and Lemon, Rose, and Poppy Seed Muffin (see page 92)
Lunch: Quinoa Bowl with Veggies (see page 80)
Snack: Grain-free Blueberry Pop Tart (see page 90) and Digestive Rose Tea (see page 101)
Dinner: Turmeric Patty Sandwich with Mint and Cilantro Dressing (see page 71)
Dessert: Raw Cookie Dough Bite (see page 95)
Night cap: Adaptogenic Beauty Milk (see page 106)

DAY 6

Morning beverage: Drink 1½–3¾ cups (350–900 ml) Warm Water with Fresh Lemon Juice (see page 52) first thing in the morning
Breakfast: Celery Juice Elixir (see page 53) and Beauty Breakfast Pudding (see page 68)
Snack: Logan's Tropical Smoothie (see page 72)
Lunch: Turmeric Patty Sandwich with Mint and Cilantro Dressing (see page 71)
Snack: Cucumber and Dill Hummus (see page 72) with celery sticks and Digestive Rose Tea (see page 101)
Dinner: Quinoa Bowl with Veggies (see page 80)
Dessert: Anandi's Ananda Raw Chocolate (see page 86)
Night cap: Adaptogenic Beauty Milk (see page 106)

DAY 7

Morning beverage: Drink 1½–3¾ cups (350–900 ml) Warm Water with Fresh Lemon Juice (see page 52) first thing in the morning
Breakfast: Celery Juice Elixir (see page 53) and warm oat bran with coconut milk
Snack: Cucumber slices with Cucumber and Dill Hummus (see page 72)
Lunch: Savory Oat Bowl (see page 83)
Snack: Lavender and Coconut Cookie (see page 93) and Digestive Rose Tea (see page 101)
Dinner: Turmeric Patty Sandwich with Mint and Cilantro Dressing (see page 71) with mixed salad greens dressed with lemon juice
Dessert: Grain-free Adaptogenic Chocolate Nougat Bar (see page 89)
Night cap: Adaptogenic Beauty Milk (see page 106)

DAY 4

Morning beverage: Drink 1½–3¾ cups (350–900 ml) Warm Water with Fresh Lemon Juice with raw honey (see page 52) first thing in the morning
Breakfast: Deep Chocolate Elixir (see page 108) and Lemon, Rose, and Poppy Seed Muffin (see page 92)
Lunch: Lemon and Thyme Potatoes with Mixed Salad Greens (see page 76) and Weight-loss Tea (see page 99)
Dinner: Steamed kale and carrots with grated fresh ginger in a low-sodium vegetable broth
Dessert: Anandi's Ananda Raw Chocolate (see page 86)
Night cap: Saffron and Lemon Elixir (see page 101)

DAY 5

Morning beverage: Drink 1½–3¾ cups (350–900 ml) Warm Water with Fresh Lemon Juice with raw honey (see page 52) first thing in the morning
Breakfast: Spring Herbed Frittata (see page 75) and Weight-loss Tea (see page 99)
Lunch: Beautifying Guacamole (see page 79) with mixed salad greens and steamed broccoli
Dinner: Grain-free Orange Zest Pancakes (see page 96)
Dessert: Raw Cookie Dough Bite (see page 95)
Night cap: Saffron and Lemon Elixir (see page 101)

DAY 6

Morning beverage: Drink 1½–3¾ cups (350–900 ml) Warm Water with Fresh Lemon Juice with raw honey (see page 52) first thing in the morning
Breakfast: Lala's Detox Smoothie (see page 79)
Lunch: Lemon and Thyme Potatoes with Mixed Salad Greens (see page 76) and Weight-loss Tea (see page 99)
Dinner: Two Turmeric Patties (see page 71–without the dressing, bun, or lettuce) with cooked quinoa and mixed salad greens dressed with lemon juice
Dessert: Grain-free Adaptogenic Chocolate Nougat Bar (see page 89)
Night cap: Saffron and Lemon Elixir (see page 101)

DAY 7

Morning beverage: Drink 1½–3¾ cups (350–900 ml) Warm Water with Fresh Lemon Juice with raw honey (see page 52) first thing in the morning
Breakfast: Deep Chocolate Elixir (see page 108) and Lemon, Rose, and Poppy Seed Muffin (see page 92)
Lunch: Chickpea Pasta with Cashew Cream Sauce (see page 85) with mixed salad greens and steamed zucchini (courgettes) and Weight-loss Tea (see page 99)
Dinner: Beautifying Guacamole (see page 79) with mixed salad greens and steamed zucchini (courgette)
Dessert: Raw Cookie Dough Bite (see page 95)
Night cap: Saffron and Lemon Elixir (see page 101)

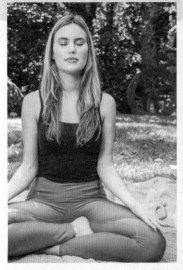

When we slow down and
simplify all that we are doing,
we can begin to see clearly
what is needed.

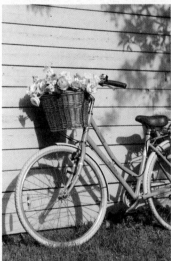

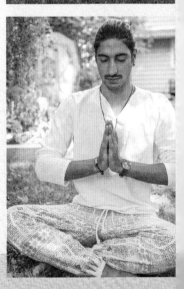

chapter 4

MOVEMENT: SIMPLE YOGA AND BREATHING PRACTICES

Yoga is one of the most important aspects of Ayurveda. In this chapter, you will learn how to move your body, how to connect to yourself, how to use your breath, and simple practices to squeeze in during your busy day to keep your body thriving.

Prana: How to Maximize Your Breath and Breathe Better

I know it seems pretty obvious to say that we need to breathe in order to live, but did you know you can use your breath to maximize your life span, combat stress, and manipulate the energetic flow in your body?

The Sanskrit word *prana* means both "life-force energy" and "breath;" it doesn't have a single direct translation or function. When we talk about prana in Ayurveda, we are talking about giving more life to the body, mind, and spirit on a subtle level. Prana is the root source of all the energy in the universe. All forces of nature are manifestations of prana. Think about your breath as a subtle force that not only fills your physical body with life-giving energetic oxygen but also fills your mind and emotional body with energetic vitality. When we inhale deeply and consciously, we breathing oxygen into our lungs as well as taking in the environment and knowledge found in all of life.

Prana is the driving force behind all things. It is prana that keeps things moving in and around us. Without prana, life is gray, dark, cloudy, and full of stagnant energy. With prana, life is bright, creative, open, full, loving, and flowing. Prana can be found in the food we eat, the liquid we drink, the air we breathe, the warmth of the sun, and the people and places around us. This is why relationships feel so good, we are transferring this pranic energy from person to person.

Ayurveda teaches that illness and symptoms of sickness are clear manifestations of obstructed or decreased pranic flow. If you aren't sure of how to begin healing yourself, a good place to start is by practicing conscious breathing. What does it mean to be conscious of your breath? It means that you are aware of your own inhale/exhale and you can feel the energy of the air flowing in and out of your body.

So, are you getting all of the prana you deserve? Answer the following questions as honestly as possible:

- Am I using my breath wisely?
- Am I gaining energy from the air I breathe, the food I eat, and the relationships I have?
- Do I utilize my full lung capacity?
- Am I aware of my surroundings?
- Do I gain strength from my breath?
- Do I deplete my energy with activities or people?
- Am I draining the energy of other people with my own energy?
- Is my life stressful and chaotic?
- Am I able to redirect negative energy into positive feelings?
- Is it hard for me to focus?
- Do I waste a lot of time and procrastinate daily?
- Are my thoughts, actions, and words overly self-critical and negative?

These questions are intended to help you see where you are on your journey, what areas you can improve upon, and where any imbalances may lie.

Simple Breathing Exercise to Increase Prana and Release Stress

This exercise is called a pranic breath. Start with one pranic breath and work your way up (in your own time) to ten. Do this practice at least once a day.

- Sit comfortably, cross-legged on the floor, if possible. You can use a bolster or blankets to prop your legs up or lean against a wall to help you sit up tall. Try to relax your shoulders, allowing your shoulder blades to roll down your back toward your waist. This will help to lift your chest up and create space for your ribcage to move freely.
- Place your palms together in front of your heart. Push with pressure against both palms to create an activation of energy between both spheres of the body.
- Gently close your lips and focus only on breathing through your nose.
- Inhale for the count of ten, breathing in deeply though your nose and drawing your breath down into your lungs. Feel the breath expanding in your ribcage and trickling down into your belly, expanding deeper and wider. Imagine this breath as a golden white light that is pulling in all of Mother Nature's beautiful invigorating energy and sucking it deep into your body.

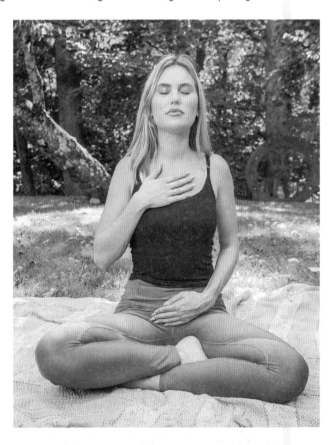

- Once your lungs and belly are full of this life-giving air, hold your breath for the count of ten (or as long as possible). Focus all of this energy to your third eye (the middle point in between your eyebrows). Imagine this space filling with all the golden white light that is building and swirling with prana.
- Exhale for the count of ten. As you slowly exhale, imagine the golden white light showering over your whole body and leaving you energized and with all your senses vital.

Ayurveda and Yoga: How to Move for Your Dosha

Ayurveda is not just about eating for your mind-body type but also heavily incorporates lifestyle practices like movement. Yoga is a sister science to Ayurveda, which is why it is the recommended type of movement for the lifestyle you are building. It's not necessary for you to get intensely into yoga if it's not in alignment with what you like; you can apply the ideals of the suggested movements to any other type of movement you like.

Best Yoga Poses for Vata

Since people with a Vata constitution are prone to anxiety, overexhaustion, and fatigue, the best thing to do is combat those symptoms with the opposite energetics. Vatas are highly energetic and erratic in nature, which is why it is recommended that they

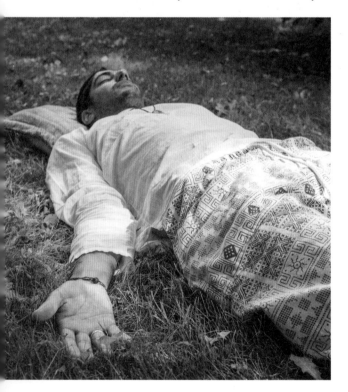

move their bodies to help calm and ground themselves. The best way to do this is with slow-moving yoga poses that reduce anxiety and stress. Fast-paced yoga flows will aggravate Vata in the long term (if not immediately).

If you are participating in a high-energy activity or style of yoga, I suggest you slow down the movement and take long pauses and breaks to offset what you are doing. Your body will love and thrive with restorative yoga, yin yoga, and extended practice of the Corpse Pose (see right) for about twenty minutes.

IMPORTANT

For all of the following poses, use your prana-enhancing yoga breath: breathe in through your nose and out through your nose.

Corpse Pose (*Savasana*)

Benefits: Repairs tissues and rejuvenates cells, relaxes muscles, improves breathing, and helps enhance meditation for those with an active mind.

- Lie flat on the floor with your back connected to the ground and your arms relaxed by your sides, palms facing up. Your legs can be more than hip-width apart. Let your legs and feet roll out, letting go of any tension. This pose is about relaxation and slowing down.
- Focus on your breath and let your thoughts come and go, sending breath and a healing light to each thought.
- Slowly relax every muscle and nerve of your body, relaxing and releasing into the floor. Stay here and just breathe.
- To come out of the pose, slowly wiggle your fingers and toes and wake up each part of your body before you decide to roll over and sit up.

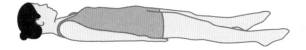

Mountain Pose (*Tadasana*)

Benefits: Reduces anxiety and stress while grounding you to your root.

- Stand with your arms at your sides. Roll your shoulders down your spine, releasing any tension in your head, neck, or shoulders. Distribute your weight evenly across both feet. Imagine being anchored and grounded by a string that starts at the top of your head and extends through your body, running equally down through both your inner ankles, outer ankles, big toes, and little toes.
- Breathe in through your nose and out through your nose. Stay in Mountain Pose for two minutes.

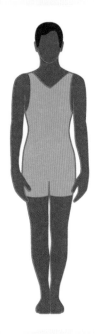

Tree Pose (*Vrksasana*)

Benefits: Helps to build strength while grounding and rooting you to the earth.

- Stand in Mountain Pose (see page 119). Shift your weight onto your left foot and begin to bend your right knee and lift your right foot off the floor. Using your core to keep your balance, reach down and clasp your right inner ankle. Draw your right foot alongside your left inner thigh. If this is too advanced, rest your right foot on the inside of your left calf or just below the knee–do not rest your foot directly on the knee.
- Once you have gained your balance, shift your position so the center of your pelvis is directly over your left foot. Adjust your hips so your right hip and left hip are aligned. Rest your hands on your hips or, if you prefer, you can place them in front of your heart, palms pressing against each other in prayer position.
- Once you are comfortable, extend your arms above your head with palms and fingers facing each other and then press them together in prayer position. To help you keep your balance, fix your gaze on an unmoving object or spot; this will help you to remain centered and keep the energy connected to the earth. Hold this pose for as long as possible or up to five minutes.
- To come out of the pose, guide your ankle and foot back into Mountain Pose. Repeat on the other side.

Additional Practices for Vata

People with a Vata constitution are prone to constipation. Since this is a common issue for most Vatas, poses and movements that include compression of the pelvis are very healing. Simple movements to help encourage the downward flow of energy are Forward Fold (see page 127), which can be done standing or sitting, and Seated Spinal Twist (see page 127). These movements help activate the lower back and thighs, which are major regions of Vata.

Best Yoga Poses for Pitta

People with a Pitta constitution may be drawn to high-intensity sports and activities but this will inevitably throw Pitta out of balance. Pittas should cultivate a calm, relaxing, and non-competitive movement routine. Although you may find it difficult to resist the urge to compete with others in your class or at the gym, be as gentle as possible with yourself. Since you don't want to add more heat to the already fiery Pitta, it's best to avoid hot yoga, hot Pilates, boxing, running in hot weather, and any other type of movement that could cause profuse sweating. If you find that even light stretching causes you to start sweating a lot, try to practice before sunrise or after sunset–the cooler times of days. Focus on activities that are calming and cooling to the body such as taking walks barefoot through the grass in cool weather, swimming, surfing, snowboarding, and gentle yoga and use heart- and hip-opening poses to release any trapped heat in the body.

Bow Pose (*Dhanurasana*)

Benefits: Helps to open up the heart center, releasing any stagnant or trapped heat.

- Lie face-down on the floor with your arms relaxed by your sides, palms facing up. Bend your knees and exhale, bringing your heels toward your butt. Focus on sending the heels as close to your butt as possible. Make sure that your knees are hip-width apart (the distance will vary from person to person). Reach back with both hands and clasp your ankles, making sure you are holding onto your ankles and not your feet.
- On the inhale, strongly push the energy from your torso up and back, lifting your heels away from your butt and your thighs away from the floor. Your head, neck, torso, and shoulders should be off the floor. You should feel the back bend at this point. Don't tighten your back muscles.
- Softly send the inhale and exhale into your chest, releasing any tension and gently rolling your shoulders down and back to open your heart even more. Breathe into your back as breathing may be slightly difficult with the pressure of your body on your belly. Don't hold your breath; the breath helps you open and stretch into tight areas of the body to release pain and heat. Try to stay in this pose for twenty seconds.
- To come out of the pose, release on the exhale and relax your body, head turned to the left, hands folded under your face. Lie quietly for a minute. Repeat two more times.

Fish Pose (*Matsyasana*)

Benefits: Strengthens the upper back muscles and stretches the front of the body and hip flexors.

- Lie flat on your back with both legs extended straight in front of your body and your arms relaxed by your sides, palms facing down.
- Press both forearms and elbows into the floor, lifting your chest upward to the sky and creating a slight arch in your upper back. The goal is to create an arch in your upper back in order to release tension in the chest.
- Tilt your head back toward the floor and place the crown of your head on the floor. (If your head does not reach the floor or you need more support, use a yoga block, bolster, or blanket to support the back of your head.) This will draw the energy of your shoulder blades down and back and lift your upper torso off the floor. Use your forearms and hands to stabilize your body and keep the pressure off your head. Press upward through your heels to keep your thighs engaged and active.

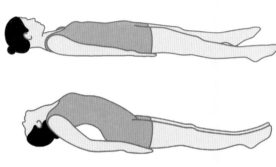

- Inhale and exhale for ten breaths, holding for five at the top of each breath.
- To come out of the pose, press firmly into your forearms, allowing your head to release off the floor. Exhale, bring your torso to the floor and draw your knees up and in toward your chest. Wrap your arms around your knees and give them a hug. Relax and repeat two more times.

Additional Practices for Pitta

People with a Pitta constitution benefit greatly from meditation and earthing. Earthing is the practice of connecting with the earth by walking barefoot across it, which helps to cool and calm the body. Try to do a walking meditation around your yard, block, or somewhere outside your home for at least ten minutes once a day at sun down. You don't only have to walk across grass to feel the earth, walking on pavement or cement might feel weird at first but this is an effective form of earthing as well. Focus on your breathing, release your thoughts, and connect your body to the earth.

Best Yoga Poses for Kapha

People with a Kapha constitution have the most stamina and strength of the three doshas but they love to be sedentary. They are so grounded that they don't even want to move, which is the exact reason why Kaphas need to do invigorating, warm, and fast-paced yoga or other activities.

Kaphas who are out of balance experience severe lethargy, weight gain, and depression, which is why movement is their medicine. Exercise not only helps to invigorate a Kapha's energy but also releases endorphins that combat mood swings and depression. Kickboxing, high-intensity interval training (HIIT), hot Pilates, and warm infrared yoga are all optimal for Kaphas. If you tend to be sluggish in the morning, try to get your movement in between the hours of 6 a.m. and 10 a.m. as this will help sustain an energized state and keep you motivated throughout the day.

Downward-facing Dog (*Adho Mukha Svanasana*)

Benefits: Helps to energize the entire body and rev up cardiovascular energy, which will get the heat moving throughout the body.

- Kneel on a yoga mat with your knees hip-width apart, your arms straight, and your palms on the floor. Spread your palms wide and stack your shoulders over your wrists. This is Table-top Pose. You will need to keep your knees hip-width apart throughout the entire pose.
- When you're comfortable, curl your toes under and lift your knees off the ground. Raise your body up, lifting from your pelvis, and straighten your legs. Press down to send the energy out of your heels and try to place both heels on the yoga mat. You may need to readjust your arms and walk the palms of your hands out in front of your shoulders slightly.

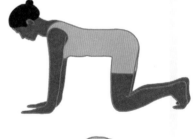

- Imagine a string pulling your belly toward your back, breathe deeply, and hold the inverted V position. Stay in this pose for twenty breaths.
- To come out of the pose, bend your knees and fold back into Table-top Pose.

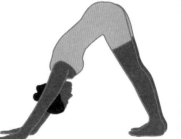

Downward-facing Dog (*Adho Mukha Svanasana*) to Plank Position (*Kumbhakasana*)

Benefits: Builds core and upper body strength (but if you struggle with Plank Position, holding Downward-facing Dog for an extended period will also build your core and upper body strength).

- Starting from Downward-facing Dog (see page 123), inhale and draw your torso forward until your arms are perpendicular (at right angles) to the floor and your shoulders are directly over your wrists. Your torso should be parallel to the floor, as if you were doing a push-up. Resist your butt going up toward the ceiling and lengthen your tailbone back toward your heels. Lift your head up and look straight down at the floor, keeping the back of your neck relaxed and your throat soft.
- Once you are comfortable in Plank Position, roll back and forth from Plank to Downward-facing Dog, increasing your pace and bringing up your heart rate. Do this for two minutes straight, no break.

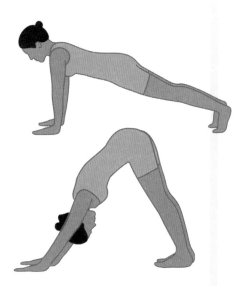

Additional Practices for Kapha

Kaphas need and thrive with daily movement. If yoga is not your favorite form of exercise, find a physical hobby that you love and do it daily. Biking, dancing, and running are great alternatives. Even a swift morning walk is enough to get Kapha moving. If you find yourself wanting to be more sedentary for no apparent reason, this is a sign that Kapha is out of balance and you need to up your daily movement.

Self-love and Movement:
How to Stay Active Every Day

It's difficult to stay active and move your body daily when you are busy taking care of kids, working long hours at a desk, spending time with family, or just overall trying to do it all. However, movement is vital for your health (not just your physical health but also your mental health), so instead of looking at movement—whether it be yoga, the gym, sports, dance, classes, etc.–as a chore, try thinking about moving your body as a form of self-love. The more we love ourselves, the more we thrive.

Every day you have an opportunity to honor your body by nourishing it, moving it, and loving it. When you stay active and keep your body moving in an organic way that is a natural complement to the energetics of your body, you will find that life flows with more ease and less stress. Movement is a huge part of longevity and living a balanced life. When you move your body you are treating yourself with the respect you deserve. Your body deserves to be treated right 100 percent of the time.

You may find it difficult to stay motivated when it comes to daily movement but doing at least ten minutes of designated yoga or any other activity will really help your mind-body connection and create more space for healing.

Movement can be done anywhere, at any time; every little bit you do counts! Here are five ways to stay active:

- **Stretch, dance, jump around, and move as soon as you wake up in the morning:** Five minutes is all you need. This not only gets your energy up for the day but also wakes up all your body parts.
- **Walk or bike to work:** Doing some movement before you start work will increase your focus and prolong your energy. If your work is too far away to walk or bike, park your car further away from your place of work and walk the longest distance possible to get there.
- **Stop, drop, and stretch:** Try to take a two-minute break from work every hour to move your body in an organic way. This will help you feel motivated and ready to work again. You don't only have to stretch, you could do push-ups, crunches, squats, planks, dance, whatever feels right to you.
- **Take a break:** Whether you work from home or elsewhere, you can add movement into your post-lunchtime routine. Light movement, like walking, is helpful for digestion after you have eaten. Either walk to a park to eat your lunch and then walk back or take a walk around the block after you eat. If you live in a very cold climate and work in an office, just take a walk up and down the stairs if you don't want to go outdoors.
- **Do activities with friends:** It's much easier to stay motivated when you have a partner to help keep you accountable. Suggest going for a walk instead of meeting for tea to chat. Instead of going out to a bar, go to a salsa or Zumba class and shake your hips. There are plenty of fun activities you can do with others that will keep you connected while moving together.

Daily Routine: Asanas for Anywhere

Here are a few asanas (poses) you can do anywhere, any time. These simple practices can release stress, improve mobility, promote healthy circulation throughout the body, open up energy in the lower spine, massage internal organs, and aid digestion.

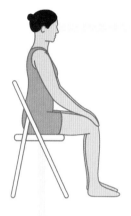

Spinal Flex

This pose is great for anyone who does little to no movement during their day, particularly those who are stuck behind a desk all day or who spend all their time driving around in a car. You don't even have to get up! You may do the Spinal Flex as a five-minute break throughout the day.

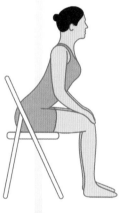

- Sit in your chair with a straight spine. Place both feet flat on the floor, about hip-width apart. Place your right hand on your right knee and your left hand on your left knee. Your arms should be activated but not stiff.

- Begin breathing in and out of your nose, filling your belly with each breath and releasing and pushing your navel to your spine. On the inhale, focus on filling your entire diaphragm. On the exhale, try pushing your breath to the back of your throat and down. (The exhale should sound like a hiss). It's okay if you don't get the breath right the first couple of times, with practice, it will come. It is essential to create an internal awareness during yoga, not only to reap the greatest benefits but also to prevent injury to the body.

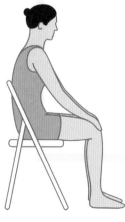

- With each inhale, arch your spine forward, lifting your heart space upward and pulling your shoulders open and back. Keep your head still and shoulders relaxed. With each exhale, focus on pushing the breath out of your body while arching your spine back in the shape of a C. Roll your shoulders forward and tuck your navel toward your spine. Do this five times or as many times as you need to feel relaxed and tension free.

Seated Spinal Twist (*Marichyasana III*)

Twisting the spine has many benefits. It massages the abdominal muscles and organs, promoting digestion, and keeps the spine healthy. The spine builds up tension between the vertebrae that can cause stagnation and when we twist the spine we release the hidden tension. This is a wonderful pose, especially for Vatas, because it helps move energy downward.

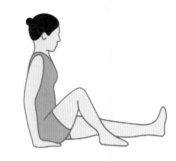

- Sit on the floor with your left leg outstretched and your right leg bent at the knee with your right foot on the floor. I lift my butt cheeks and push them to the side so I can really feel my sit bones—this helps to lengthen the spine.
- Inhale, raising your arms up to lengthen your spine and twisting to the right toward the bent thigh, compressing your belly against the thigh. Allow your right hand to rest behind you as if it's a support for keeping your spine straight—you don't want to hunch over. Press your left elbow into the right thigh to increase the stretch.

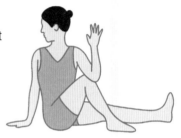

- If you feel comfortable, turn your neck toward the back of your right shoulder and allow your gaze to follow. Hold for five breaths. Repeat on the other side.

Seated Forward Fold (*Paschimottanasana*)

Every day I see clients who complain of back pain and intense lower back tightness. One of the easiest methods of relief for back pain is a Seated Forward Fold.

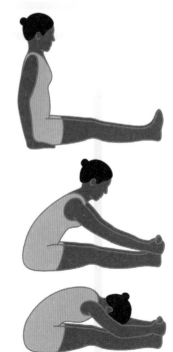

- Sit on the floor with your legs stretched out in front of you. Make sure you can feel your sit bones under you and that you are balanced and sitting up tall.
- Inhale, raising your arms up toward the sky and extending them as long as you can.
- On the exhale, lift from your chest and fold forward from your hips toward your toes. Keep your chest lifted to protect your spine; don't collapse. If you can't reach your toes, that's okay, touch wherever you can: ankles, knees, thighs. If this is uncomfortable and your hamstrings are too tight, you can practice this pose using a blanket or yoga block under your tailbone. Hold the pose for five breaths and repeat as needed.

I embody love in its truest form. Everything I see is an act of love or a call for love. I honor the dark in others and shed light upon them. I choose to follow love and release fear. I choose to infuse love into negative situations that tempt me with doubt. I trust in love and I claim peace and happiness within.

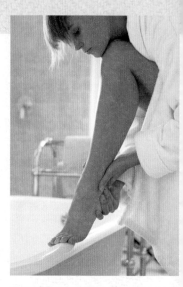

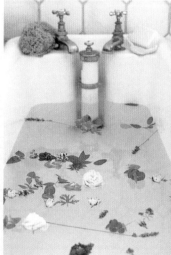

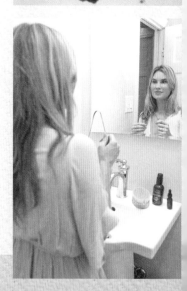

chapter 5

SELF-LOVE PRACTICES: TAKE TIME FOR YOURSELF

The stagnation of energy, toxins, and emotions can back us up and weigh us down. In this chapter, I will teach you how to make time for yourself. You will learn how to treat yourself with the daily love, respect, and nourishment that you deserve. Incorporating practices such as self-massage, bathing rituals, positive thought patterns, mantras, beauty treatments, moon rituals, and essential oils will enhance your path to wellness. Give yourself permission to open your heart and feel. Untie the weight of stagnation, release it back into the earth, and cleanse your spirit.

Anoint: Give Back to Your Body with Essential Oils and Aromatherapy

Essential oils can help to heal your emotional and physical bodies, which makes aromatherapy a wonderful tool to add to your self-healing kit. It is easy to incorporate the sacred act of anointing yourself with this potent form of medicine into your daily life. I take my oils with me wherever I go so I can stop and anoint myself whenever I'm in stressful situations, lacking focus, in need of a pick-me-up, or want to relax.

You may notice that you are drawn to a specific scent. If you are called to a particular oil, this may hold some significance to what you are going through at that time. For example, when I go through trauma, I tend to gravitate toward the scent of lavender. During the worst of my illness, I carried

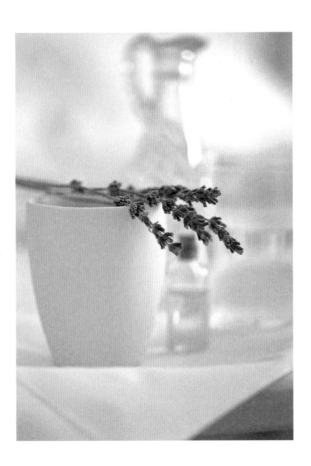

Caution

- Always test oils on a small patch of your skin to ensure you are not allergic before applying them to the rest of your body.
- Some essential oils are not suitable for use during pregnancy or for use on babies and children. Never use essential oils internally and avoid direct use on the skin. Some oils can cause photosensitivity. Always read the label and contact a specialist if you need more guidance.
- Some essential oils are better for us than others. It's important to know the quality of your oils and never ingest any that are not food grade. (See page 156 for recommendations.)

lavender oil with me everywhere I went. Lavender is calming and soothing to the nerves, and also pacifies anxiety.

You can add essential oils to your bathwater, use them to make your own room fresheners and perfumes, or apply diluted oils to your body. To use essential oils on your body, add a few drops of the essential oil to a carrier oil (such as olive oil) and then place a drop of the combined oil on your temples, your pulse points, or the soles of your feet, or behind your ears. You could also simply add a few drops to a cloth and inhale.

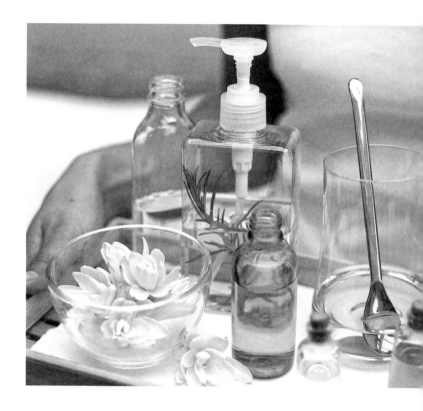

The Best Essential Oils for Your Dosha

VATA Since Vata is associated with Air and Ether, the best oils for people with a Vata constitution are warming and grounding. I suggest patchouli, rose geranium, palo santo, lavender, sage, cedar, vanilla, basil, and amber.

PITTA When you have a pitta imbalance or notice your fiery energy coming out, choose cooling and calming oils. I recommend jasmine, lavender, mint, peppermint, gardenia, chamomile, ylang-ylang, and sandalwood.

KAPHA People who have a high amount or imbalance of Kapha tend to need more invigorating scents and a boost of energy. I suggest sweet orange, eucalyptus, ginger, juniper, clove, and cinnamon.

Self-massage: The Art of Abhyanga

The Sanskrit word *abhyanga* means "oil massage." Abhyanga is a form of massage that is viewed as a medicinal therapy. It's been shown to provide deep nourishing and cleansing effects on the entire bodily system.

Traditionally, this lymphatic massage is performed by two practitioners working in sync with each other. However, the practice can also be performed as a self-massage, which is just as beneficial and is considered to be one of the highest forms of healing.

Abhyanga is done by massaging warm herbal oil onto the entire body before bathing. It helps to nourish the tissues of the body; stimulates the organs; increases circulation; slows down aging; brings longevity; balances all three doshas; softens, clears, and increases firmness of the skin; helps combat insomnia; detoxes the lymphatic system;

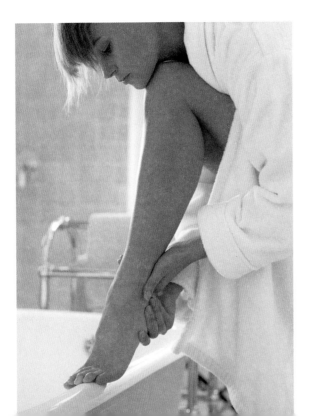

Oil Pulling

Oil pulling is an Ayurvedic technique to remove toxins from the blood. It involves swishing a tablespoon of oil in your mouth on an empty stomach for around 20 minutes. (It takes 20 minutes for our blood to circulate out of the heart, through our bodies, and back to the heart.) You shouldn't swallow the oil. You can start practicing oil-pulling for just 5 minutes at a time and work your way up to 20 minutes. Always brush your teeth after oil-pulling.

The benefits of oil-pulling include detoxification of the mouth tissues, healing inflamed or bleeding gums, whitening and strengthening teeth, removing plaque, and boosting immunity. It's wonderful to do oil-pulling during self-massage or in the shower.

and clears the channels of the body. The heat of the massage stimulates neuropeptides in the skin and nourishes the body on a cellular level. Neuropeptides –small protein-like molecules–help neurons communicate with each other in specific ways. In the case of abhyanga, these neuropeptides stimulate the communication to heal the body.

The Best Base Oils for Your Dosha

The quality of the oil you use to massage your body matters. Avoid using low-quality and/or rancid oils because your skin will absorb every bit of any product you put on it.

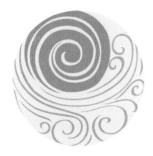

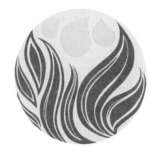

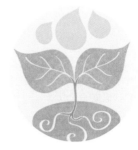

VATA One of the more unstable elements, Vata needs extra nourishment. If your constitution is predominately Vata or you live in a cool, dry climate and notice you have extra-dry or cracked skin, the practice of abhyanga can strengthen your tissues on a cellular level. I recommend using cold-pressed sesame oil. Sesame oil is heavy and lubricating, which helps to balance and calm the cold dryness that Vata can present.

PITTA Individuals with a Pitta nature have no problem producing extra heat, which means a lighter, more cooling oil is going to be optimal for those with a predominately Pitta constitution or who live in warmer climates. I recommend using a cold-pressed coconut or sunflower oil. A mixture of the two oils can provide a nice balance as well. Both oils are light and cooling, which helps to soothe, cleanse, and relax an overly heated and tense Pitta person.

KAPHA People with a Kapha nature tend to need stimulation and invigorating energy to keep balance. If you have a predominantly Kapha dosha or live in a cool, wet climate, choosing a light and warming oil will be the best option. Massaging with a mix of cold-pressed sunflower and sesame oil will give Kapha the right amount of warmth without being too heavy. Massaging with this combination will stimulate the Earth element in Kapha, bringing vital energy to all limbs.

ALL THREE DOSHAS

Jojoba oil has the potent energetics to balance Vata, Pitta, and Kapha. It is the perfect tri-doshic oil.

How to Perform Self-massage

I recommend doing self-abhyanga daily. Here is an easy step-by-step guide to help you incorporate this ancient practice into your everyday self-care routine. The massage starts at the top of your head and works its way down the front and back of your body. You can oil just the top of your scalp or you may choose to oil your entire head, including your hair.

Remember to always test oils on a small patch of your skin to ensure you are not allergic before you apply the oil all over your body.

4–8 fl oz (120–250 ml) massage oil

heat-safe container, such as a ceramic, glass, or bpa-free plastic bowl

old towel

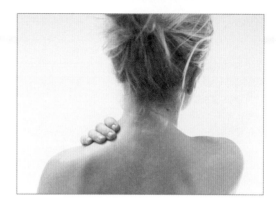

1   Warm the oil in a heat-safe container to a little warmer than body temperature. (I like to warm the oil in a double boiler/bain-marie on the stove so I can manage the temperature more efficiently. You may also heat the oil in the microwave in 30-second increments, testing the temperature as you go.) To test the temperature of the oil, carefully apply a small spot of oil to your wrist to make sure it is not too hot.

2   Stand on an old towel in your bathroom–the towel will catch any excess oil so it doesn't stick to the floor.

3   Pour some oil into the palms of your hands, the more oil the better! Cover your entire body with the oil.

4   Using small circular strokes, massage the crown of your head. If you don't want oil in your hair, begin the massage at your ears. Avoid using the oil on your face, except for your ears and neck.

5   Using upward strokes and an open hand to create friction, massage the front and back of your neck.

6   Using a clockwise circular motion, massage around your breasts/chest.

7   Using a clockwise circular motion, massage your stomach/abdominal area. You really need to work in deep here. If you are pregnant,

HOW TO MAKE YOUR OWN SELF-MASSAGE OIL

To enhance your abhyanga, you can add essential oils specific to your dosha (see page 131) to your recommended base oil (see page 133). Add 10–20 drops of your preferred essential oil–you can mix different ones together if you like–to a 12-fl-oz (350-ml) container of your dosha-specific base oil.

recovering from surgery, or have chronic pain in this area, consult your specialist before deeply massaging the area.

8 Using long up and down strokes, rub one of your arms to create friction and heat. Once you have created heat, massage the entire arm with a circular motion, starting at the bottom of the wrist and working upward toward the heart on the inside of the arm. Repeat on the other arm.

9 Add some extra oil to your hands and, without straining, reach around to your back and spine and gently massage with up and down strokes.

10 Vigorously massage up and down your legs up to create friction and heat. Focus on the top of one thigh and work your way down the leg, taking care to work your hands in a circular motion on the insides of your legs (this is a huge lymphatic part and many toxins build up in these areas). Repeat on the other leg.

11 Take some extra time to focus on your feet. Really work the oil into your feet and don't leave a single toe untouched.

12 Once you've finished the massage, take a warm shower or bath for as long as feels comfortable. The idea is to open the pores to let the oil sink in deeper. Don't use soap to wash off the oil (it's not necessary). Towel dry after you shower or bathe. Take caution when stepping out of the bathtub or shower, as the floor may be slippery.

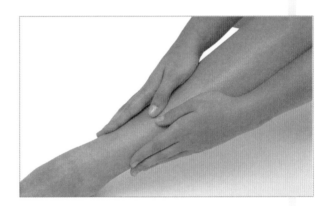

Adapting Self-Massage for Your Dosha

VATA Use a slower pace to help keep you calm and grounded.

PITTA Use a moderate pace and circular motions rather than friction to keep heat at a minimum.

KAPHA Use swift and powerful friction to move excess tissue and toxins to the blood for detox.

Bathe: Turn Your Bathroom into a Sanctuary

Taking a bath is deeply therapeutic, providing benefits for both your mind and body. In ancient times, bathing was revered as a holy act of self-love. Turning your bathroom into a peaceful sanctuary is an easy way to slow down, bring love into your life, and treat your physical and emotional body with kindness.

A clean bathroom is just as important as a clean body. When we clean our bodies, we feel lighter, more balanced, and achieve a sense of clarity; the same goes for cleaning the spaces we live and function in. It is optimal to use all-natural, chemical-free cleaning supplies when setting the tone for your sacred space. (See page 156 for recommendations.)

Aside from physically cleaning your space, you can take the process one step further and do a simple energy cleanse using either sage or palo santo smudge sticks (see page 157), which both cleanse stagnant energy and smell wonderful. Sage and palo santo have both been used for centuries to ward off negative people, emotions, situations, and energy. If you have lots of people coming in and out of your bathroom on a daily basis, cleansing the room is a good step to take so you can really heal in your sacred space and avoid picking up anyone else's energetic baggage.

How to Do a Simple Energy Cleanse

- Carefully light a sage or palo santo smudge stick, let it burn until you see smoke, and then blow the flame out.
- Waft the smoke around the outline of your body (being careful not to touch yourself) and in the areas of your home where you wish to clear energy.
- Once you've cleansed all the desired areas of your home, open a small window and let the negative energy out.

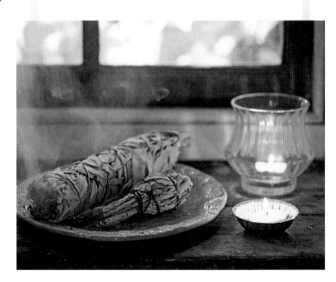

How to Use the Elements of the Earth in your Bathroom Sanctuary

Customize your bathing experience and use the following tools to enhance your bath time and create self-love rituals.

Water: Fill your bathtub with warm water–this is great for pacifying Vata. If you want to experience a detoxing effect, increase the temperature of the water. If you have a Pitta flare-up or imbalance, fill the bathtub with cool or cold water. As a rule of thumb for self-healing baths, it's best to stay in the water for as little as 20 minutes or up to 1 hour.

Sounds: Set the mood with soothing tones. (You could try using the calm app, see page 157.) Listening to the sounds of nature and different vibrational frequencies can help you tap into your more Earthy (Kapha) side. Sounds can bring feelings of relaxation or levity, and they allow us to drop our menial thoughts and help us to focus inward.

Candles: The sacred element of Fire (Pitta) can be introduced with candles. I like to use unscented candles (see page 157)–as many as possible! Put a couple of candles on the inside corner of your bathtub or just leave them on a shelf in your bathroom. Whether you take a bath in the morning, at midday, or at night, using candles will surround you with natural light instead of stimulating or tiring your eyes with artificial light bulbs. This natural light will bring ease, calm, and a sense of sacredness into your space. Important: Never leave a burning candle unattended.

Incense: A beautiful way to invoke a sense of ritual is to use incense. It has been used for centuries in prayer and offering to Higher Source. By lighting incense after you cleanse your space, you are

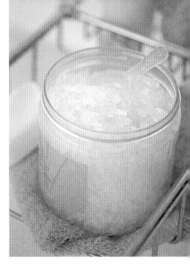

inviting positive radiant energy and spirit to fill your room.

Salt: Fill your bathtub with water and add 2–4 cups (450–900 g) mineral salts, such as sea salt or Epsom salt. Salt is known for its ability to trap negative energy and clear it from a person, space, or object. Epsom salt is the most basic and potent salt you can add to your bath. Epsom salts reduce stress, eliminate toxins, and decrease pain, inflammation, and bloat.

Essential oils: You can use essential oils to heal on an emotional and physical level (see page 131). Dry herbs, flowers, fruits, and plants can all bring us the essence of Mother Earth and help us connect to a deeper healing, as well as infusing our bathwater with heightened energetics. For example, citrus fruits are uplifting and roses evoke feelings of beauty and love. Take a dying bouquet of flowers from your home and, instead of throwing them in the trash, scatter the petals in your bathwater. For a cleansing and enlivening shower or bath, attach a bunch of eucalyptus leaves to the top of your shower head or under the bath tap before turning on the water.

Crystals: Healing crystals are a wonderful way to raise the vibration and emit positive healing energy throughout a space. Citrine or amethyst work best for Vata, amethyst or rose quartz for Pitta, and orange calcite or carnelian for Kapha.

Healing Bath Recipes to Guide You on Your Journey Toward Self-love

Customize your bathing experience and use the following tools to enhance your bath time and create self-love rituals.

Detox Bath

These bath salts help to draw toxins out of the body and soften the skin. This invigorating treatment is particularly wonderful for Kapha.

2 cups (450 g) Epsom salts

1 cup (225 g) baking soda (bicarbonate of soda)

10 drops of ginger essential oil

1 large lemon, washed and sliced

Makes enough for 1 use

Fill your bathtub with warm water and then add all the ingredients. Soak in the bath for 20 minutes–1 hour.

Rose Milk Bath

You couldn't dream up a more luxurious bath for your skin than this concoction. The lactic acid in the milk helps to remove dead skin, while the rose oil calms and tones new skin. This beauty bath is great for nourishing and taming Pitta.

1½ cups (190 g) milk powder (raw if available)

½ cup (130 g) Himalayan pink salt

1 handful dried or fresh rose petals

10 drops of rose essential oil

Makes enough for 1 use

Put all the ingredients except the rose petals in a bowl of warm water and stir until the milk powder and salt dissolve. Fill your bathtub with water, then add the milk and salt mixture and sprinkle in the rose petals. Soak in the bath for 20 minutes–1 hour.

Relaxing Chamomile Bath

As you learned in chapter 3, adaptogens (see page 59) are an amazing additive for our daily lives. Ashwagandha powder is supportive of Vata and can help calm and relax nervousness and anxiety. Magnesium flakes are crucial for the remineralization of the body and chamomile helps to ground Vata as well. The color and aroma of the flower petals, if using, will help you to reconnect your body to the earth, which also reduces the element of Air.

1 cup (225 g) magnesium flakes

10 drops of chamomile essential oil

½ cup (70 g) ashwagandha powder

1 handful fresh rose petals, lavender, chamomile, or other wild flowers (optional)

Makes enough for 1 use

Put all the ingredients except the fresh flowers, if using, in a bowl of warm water and stir until the magnesium flakes and ashwagandha powder dissolve. Fill your bathtub with water, then add the bath salts and sprinkle in the flowers, if using. Soak in the bath for 20 minutes–1 hour.

What if You Don't Have a Bathtub?

If you don't have a bathtub, you can use the same recipes above in a footbath. You can adjust the quantities of the ingredients to the amount of water you are using or make the footbath more potent by leaving the recipes as they are. Make sure the water in the footbath comes up to your ankles.

Enhance: Beauty Treatments to Care for Your Skin

Although beauty ultimately comes from the inside out, we can always do more to protect, heal, and prevent our skin from aging. I love doing at-home facials and find they not only keep my skin looking radiant, but also make my whole body feel relaxed and beautiful.

If you like, you can do a face mask with a partner or friend to help you connect with them on a deeper, more soulful level. I like to use different face masks about three or four times a week, but it's not necessary to do them more often than three times a month if you don't have the time.

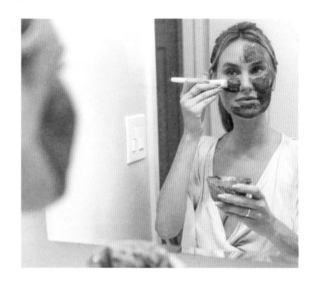

Natural Beauty Recipes

Using natural ingredients in your beauty recipes can makes the whole process of skincare more sensual. The following recipes are beneficial for all three doshas, though I've noted where some work particularly well for a specific dosha.

Moringa Mermaid Mask

Moringa powder has antiseptic qualities. It fights and heals acne, reduces inflammation, is rich in vitamin A and amino acids that help produce collagen, and balances the skin's pH. This treatment's hydrating and collagen-building effects are great for Vata.

3 tablespoons water

juice of ½ lemon

½ teaspoon pearl powder

2 tablespoons raw honey

1½ tablespoons moringa powder

Makes enough for 1–2 uses

Cleanse and dry your skin. Mix all ingredients together in a small bowl until smooth. Apply the mask to your face with your fingertips or a facial-mask brush, lightly massaging it into your skin. Leave the mask on for 15–20 minutes–lie down, walk around, or do whatever you like to do while the mask dries. Rinse off the mask with warm water.

Any leftover mask will keep for up to 4 days in an airtight container in the refrigerator. When using the mask for the second time, you may need to add a little extra water to the mixture, one drop at a time, to loosen the mask to a useable consistency.

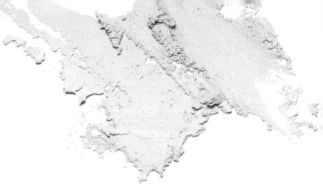

Sandalwood Shakti Mask

Nutmeg and sandalwood have been used in Ayurvedic medicine for centuries to treat rashes, inflamed skin, cystic acne, and blemishes. This is the perfect face mask for Pitta types with inflamed skin. It's also ideal for anyone who is prone to acne due to its antibacterial cooling properties.

1 tablespoon ground nutmeg

4 tablespoons whole milk (raw if available)

2 tablespoons sandalwood powder

1 tablespoon raw honey

Makes enough for 1–2 uses

Cleanse and dry your skin. Mix all the ingredients together in a small bowl until smooth. Apply the mask to your face with your fingertips or a facial-mask brush, lightly massaging it into your skin. Leave the mask on for 15– 20 minutes, lying down with a towel beneath your head so the mask doesn't drip on anything (this mask tends to be a little watery). You may feel a tingling or stinging sensation while the mask is on. That is okay, the mask is working. Rinse off the mask with cool water.

Any leftover mask will keep for up to 4 days in an airtight container in the refrigerator. When using the mask for the second time, you may need to add a little extra milk to the mixture, one drop at a time, to loosen the mask to a useable consistency.

Blossoming Beauty Mask

People with a Kapha constitution tend to have an oily and dull complexion and they often have blackheads and clogged pores. Sounds fun, right? Well, it doesn't have to be all bad. Use this exfoliating mask once or twice a week to brighten your complexion and tighten pores.

½ cup (100 g) goat milk yogurt (raw if available)

½ teaspoon rose water

1 tablespoon pink clay powder

1 tablespoon triphala powder

½ teaspoon raw honey

a spritz of Citrus-Rose Hydrosol (see opposite)

Makes enough for 1–2 uses

Cleanse and dry your skin. Mix all the ingredients together in a small bowl until smooth. Apply the mask to your face with your fingertips, lightly massaging it into your skin to give yourself a slight exfoliation. Leave the mask on for 15–20 minutes– lie down, walk around, or do whatever you like to do while the mask dries. Rinse off the mask with warm water. Mist your skin with the Citrus-Rose Hydrosol.

Any leftover mask will keep for up to 4 days in an airtight container in the refrigerator. When using the mask for the second time, you may need to add a little extra yogurt to the mixture, one drop at a time, to loosen the mask to a useable consistency.

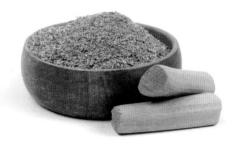

Glowing Goddess Face Oil

I created this face oil for my clients because most of them were unhappy with the results they were getting from store-bought serums and face oils. It is suitable for all skin types. You can use the face oil as a daily moisturizer, serum, or at any moment when you're in need of some self-love. I use it daily and keep it in my purse so that I can give myself a face massage whenever my skin feels dry.

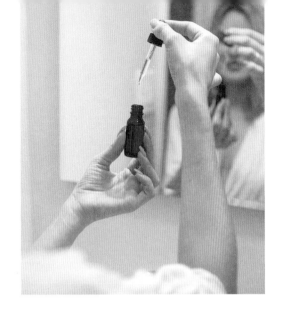

2 tablespoons jojoba oil

1 tablespoon sea buckthorn oil

1 tablespoon carrot seed oil

1 tablespoon tamanu oil

1 teaspoon rose hip oil

20–30 drops hyaluronic acid

2 drops of geranium essential oil

2 drops of frankincense essential oil

2 drops of lavender essential oil

2 drops of sandalwood essential oil

Makes about 4 fl oz (120 ml)

Mix all the ingredients together in a small bowl. Using a funnel, transfer the oil to a 4-fl-oz (120-ml) glass jar or bottle. Store in a cool, dark place. This oil will keep for up to 6 months. Massage your face daily with the oil to enhance your skin's radiance and keep it supple.

Citrus-Rose Hydrosol

A hydrosol is simply a misting moisturizer. I carry mine with me wherever I go and keep it on my bedside table because it helps me wake up and feel refreshed in the morning. It is the perfect soothing pick-me-up for your skin.

1–4 mini rose quartz crystals

½ cup (120 ml) alkaline or purified water

2 drops of colloidal silver

1 teaspoon rose water

4 drops of citrus essential oil

Makes about 4 fl oz (125 ml)

Place the rose quartz crystals at the bottom of an empty 6-fl-oz (175-ml) spray bottle, then add the remaining ingredients. Shake to mix and it's ready to spray! This hydrosol should keep for up to 1 month, or even longer if you store it in the refrigerator.

Connect: Follow the Moon's Cycles to Manifest and Clear Energy

Have you ever felt intense emotional shifts around the time of a full or new moon? The moon affects human behavior and health through its gravitational pull on bodily fluids, which is why it's important to be aware of the phases of the moon and the things you can do to help balance and clear your energy. Connecting with the moon's cycles will enhance your self-healing process and increase your awareness of your physical and emotional body. The moon represents emotions, nurturing, instinctive responses, enlightenment, and the rhythm of time.

At the Full Moon

Use the full moon as a time to give thanks for your blessings; release anything that is no longer serving you (people, items, emotions, etc.); take a cleansing bath; use palo santo smudge sticks to cleanse your ritual space (see page 136); spend

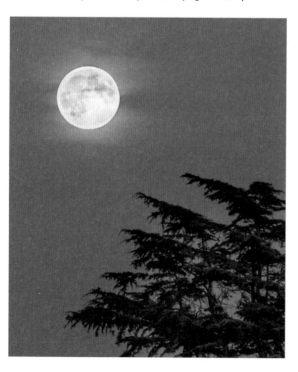

time pampering yourself to recharge; and cleanse the energy of your crystals under the light of the full moon. You could use bergamot essential oil to accompany you during this moon cycle.

At the New Moon

Use the new moon as a time to clean out the cobwebs in your life; let go of negative patterns and habits that no longer serve you; physically clean your house and personal space; meditate; and set intentions for this new cycle (focus on all the things you aspire to accomplish).

Manifest your dreams by writing them on a clean piece of paper, then speak your manifestation aloud and carry it with you throughout the cycle of the moon. When the full moon arrives, burn the paper in a fire, sending the energy up into the universe and trusting it will come into your life. You could use cypress essential oil to accompany you during this moon cycle.

Express: Let Your Voice Transform You Through Mantras

When we hide or dim our inner light from others we suffer. It's important to always speak your truth and use your voice to communicate what's inside of you. For many years, I held my words in out of fear I would be judged or received in a negative way. Although it's imperative that we are mindful of others, we need to practice being mindful of ourselves. Blurting words out is not an effective way to communicate so we need to learn new ways to navigate speaking our truth.

What is your truth? When I refer to the truth inside of you, I'm talking about the essence of you that not only makes you unique but also drives you forward on your journey. Your truth doesn't have to be your job or your career, rather it's a purposeful path that you are on, and when you stray from it you feel an innate pull back toward it.

I have used many practices to achieve the inner transformation of using my voice in a positive way. However, to avoid complicating the idea of speaking our truth in a mindful manner, I'd like to focus on a single tool: mantras.

A mantra is a sacred word, sound, sentence, or phrase that is repeated aloud or sung frequently to enhance vibration and heal the mind-body-spirit. Yogis, gurus, and similar practitioners have used mantras for centuries in the practice of meditation and transformation. Although mantras are mentioned in sacred texts throughout history, I like to take a more modern approach to the use of mantras. Anything you want to overcome, transform, change, manifest, or instill in your life can be done through the practice of singing or speaking a mantra aloud.

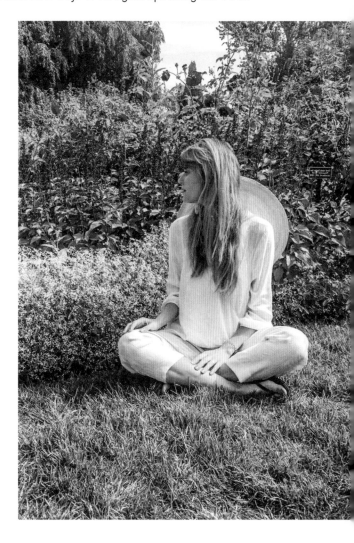

A mantra can be any saying, phrase, song, etc. that resonates with you. Exercising your voice to say what you want can have a positive effect on the way you communicate outside of your self-healing practice. The more you get used to channeling your feelings into words with clarity, the more you will begin to navigate the process of speaking your truth and communicating that truth to others. Mantras are also a wonderful way to connect with a partner or friend. Sitting in a circle or across from one another while singing a mantra can raise the vibrational energy even more.

Here are some of my favorite and most effective mantras to raise your vibration, help you cultivate clarity and confidence, and protect your energy.

- **Self-love mantra:**

  "I am confident, I am radiant,

  I am filled with joy."

- **Truth mantra:**

  "I embody my truth."

- **Protection mantra:**

  "I am safe, I am surrounded by

  light, my energy is protected."

If you would like to explore the work of using mantras more deeply, there are traditional mantras that can be sung along with music (see page 157).

How to Perform a Mantra

- Find a quiet space and sit comfortably, cross-legged on the floor or with your legs out in front of you. Become mindful of your breath, your body, and how you feel. Sit up tall and activate all the energy flowing through your body. Imagine a string tugging at the top of your head and pulling your spine upright.
- Take a few deep breaths through your nose and into your belly, exhaling through your nose. Place your hands on your heart.
- Once you have tuned into your body, mind, and spirit, begin to repeat your chosen mantra. You can either say the mantra or sing it aloud, exercising your throat chakra. Repeat the mantra aloud for at least five minutes or until you are filled with a sense of joy and the words of the mantra sing throughout your being.
- Close out this sacred practice with a prayer or blessing that you would like to be reminded of throughout the day. For example:

  "I am confident, I am radiant, I am filled with joy."

Think Positively: Affirmations to Focus on Your Goals

Positive thinking may not solve all of your problems, but negative thinking can greatly affect your outlook and reaction to life. The more you speak to yourself with negativity, the more you will suffer. Being negative is setting yourself up for failure, whereas being positive gives you an alternative route to finding happiness and peace. If you think positively, you will radiate and spread that upward energy to all areas of your life. Have you ever met someone who exudes happy energy and whose happiness just pours from their being effortlessly? If you have, that person most likely practices (on some level) shifting their energy to be more positive.

The way we think and talk to ourselves also directly affects our health. We always have a choice in life, to succumb to our woes or find new ways to overcome them. If you choose the latter, you will see the difference in your life, health, and overall happiness. However, it is important to find time to revel in your thoughts and emotions and to acknowledge your feelings and not suppress them. When we hold in our emotions, we are actually dulling our vibration and manifesting dis-ease.

Affirmations are a statement or phrase that we repeat regularly to set our intention and bring about change. They can help us stay focused on our goals. If you repeat an affirmation on a daily basis you are engraining the essence of those words inside your subconscious mind, which will help you remain positive in times of distress. I like to tape my affirmation to my bathroom mirror and I repeat it over and over again while I'm doing I'm morning routine until I'm finished.

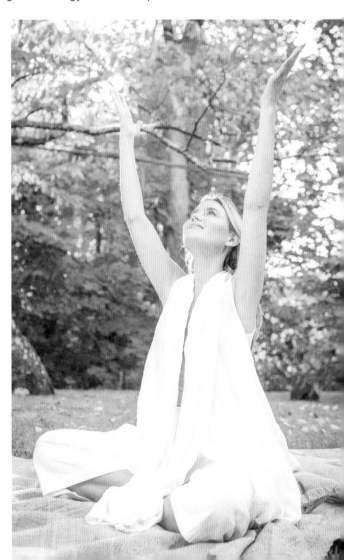

Affirmation Exercise

When your headspace feels crowded with unnecessary thoughts and your energy is low, it's time for a pick-me-up. This is a quick exercise to relieve stress, discard unwanted negative energy, and bring focus to the present moment. You can practice this anywhere, at any time. It's not necessary to sit in a meditative state but this will help in the process of shifting your thoughts and energy.

- Find a space that is safe and sacred to you and make it as comfortable as possible. Sit with your eyes open or closed.
- Breathe deeply, inhaling and exhaling through your nose for the count of five. Allow the air to fill your stomach and expand your ribcage and imagine it traveling all the way up to the top of your crown. With each inhale, visualize your breath creating a golden bubble around your body.
- Repeat this affirmation:

"My intention is to be at peace with myself; eliminate toxic feelings, elements, and energies from my life; unlearn negative and harmful practices and thought patterns; stop checking for people who don't check for me; create space for myself that is nurturing for my personal growth so that I may generate loving energy for myself and for others; nourish my spirit; and balance my energies. I have big dreams and I deserve to live a life I love and let that love radiate, today and every day I grace the Earth with my presence."

Creating Routine

Dinacharya is the Sanskrit word for "daily routine." Having a strong daily routine can help you to balance your constitution, adapt your lifestyle to your unique mind-body nature, and promote self-healing. To begin with, forming new routines can be challenging. I suggest you write out your routine and tape it to the refrigerator or a bathroom mirror so you can be reminded regularly of the things that will help you find balance.

Whenever I fall out of my routines, I immediately notice a shift in my health, usually starting with my digestion and sleep. However, when this happens, I always know that balance is awaiting me when I return to my home base and the things that bring my mind and body vitality. If you forget to incorporate some of the tools on certain days, that's okay. Don't stress, these routines are there to help guide you toward a life full of wellness, not stress you out. Remember, this is a lifelong journey and these tools will always be available to you–this is not a temporary fix, this is a lifestyle shift.

The best routines are those that are customized to an individual's way of life and particular needs. Take the morning and evening routine suggestions on pages 148–153 and apply them to your own life in a mindful way.

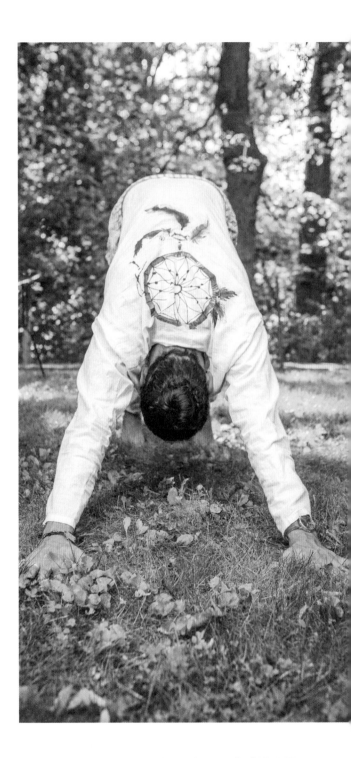

Morning Routine: The Best Rituals for Starting Your Day

Rise with the Sun

The way we begin our days sets the tone for our energy, determining how we will feel throughout the day and how well we sleep. Going to sleep early and rising early keeps our bodies on a natural cycle that helps them function at 100 percent. It's best to wake up before 6 a.m., though in the winter, when the sun rises much later, it is okay to rise before 7 a.m.. Unless you are a morning person, rising early may be a challenge for you. During the first couple of weeks, you may feel that switching your sleep schedule around is counterintuitive, but once you begin to rise early, you'll see all the ways your body and mind optimize energy throughout the day.

I always give thanks and say an internal prayer upon waking up–every new day is a blessing. Make your bed when you wake up, too.

Meditate for at Least Five Minutes

Early-morning meditation activates the bioelectric energy that helps to stimulate and direct energy to the pineal gland. The pineal gland is a pear-shaped gland in the brain that regulates hormone functions, specifically melatonin, which regulates our sleep-wake cycles. When we meditate in the morning, we are activating this system so that it can send more energy to our brains.

The act of meditation can help with focus, anxiety, mood disorders, energy levels, and overall mind-body balance. To meditate, sit in silence, focus on your breath, acknowledge any thoughts that come in to your mind and let them pass.

Without Force, Eliminate–Empty Your Bladder and Bowels

Our bodies accumulate a lot of toxins and waste while we sleep, which is why it's important to expel waste first thing in the morning. Pooping helps to cleanse the system and relieves stress from our organs.

Regular elimination is a really important function for our health. When we hold in or restrict the flow of elimination, it causes major stress on our bodies and organs. How you poop can tell you a lot about your constitution and health as well. Most people don't talk about their poop, so many people don't even know if their poop is healthy. This is a subject I talk about daily with my clients because it helps them learn about their bodies. The better you know your body, the more you can help yourself heal.

If you are prone to constipation, a morning belly massage will aid in elimination. Use the tips of your index fingers to massage the small intestines in clockwise circular motions around the navel. Repeat a rotation of these circles three to five times. Do this massage while sitting on the toilet, preferably in a squatting position. (See page 157 for details of the Squatty Potty, a foot stool that helps you to sit on the toilet in a squatting position.)

Wash Your Face

Wash your face with cool water and then gently wash your eyes with cool water as well. (Heat can build up in the eyes and cause irritation, so washing your eyes will help to keep them clear and calm.) Once you've washed your face, apply the Citrus-Rose Hydrosol (see page 141) to your skin.

Washing your face and eyes with cool water upon waking up reduces inflammation and redness and invigorates the senses. This is honestly one of the simplest acts of kindness you can do for yourself in the morning (especially if you're not a morning person). It's not actually necessary to wash your face with skincare products in the morning unless you experience night sweats and feel that your skin is extra oily. You don't want to strip your skin of its natural oil.

Brush Your Teeth and Scrape Your Tongue

This is my favorite self-care tool. Once you add this activity to your morning routine, you won't want to go a day without it. Scraping the tongue gets the body ready to digest and taste food. It also removes any ama (toxins) that have accumulated in the body overnight. It's important to remove these toxins as they may prevent the digestive system from functioning optimally.

To scrape your tongue, hold a U-shaped stainless-steel or copper tongue scraper at both long ends, place the scraper toward the back of your tongue, taking care not to hit your teeth or go too far back to your tonsils. Using mild pressure, place the edge of the scraper on the back of your tongue and scrape toward the tip of your tongue in one fluid motion. Repeat this about five times, unless you feel that it hurts, which is a sign you have already removed all the excess ama.

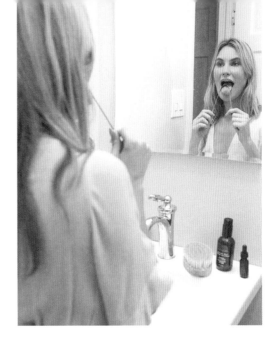

Always use a proper tongue-scraping tool; using something else, such as a spoon, could risk cutting the edge or middle of the tongue.

Drink Warm Water with Fresh Lemon Juice

Drink 1½–3¾ cups (350–900 ml) Warm Water with Fresh Lemon Juice (see page 52) in the morning. This will cleanse your bowels, promote digestion, and remove toxins. If you are not used to drinking water first thing in the morning, start with just 1 cup (250 ml) , then build up to more when your body is used to it. It's best to consume warm water throughout the day–this aids in detoxification, helps maintain a healthy weight, and keeps skin clear.

Get Moving

Start your day with movement, such as yoga, Pilates, or cycling. Stick to a type of movement that is best for your dosha (see pages 118–124). Movement doesn't have to be intense–it can be as simple as stretching or walking. Movement helps keep circulation and blood flow healthy. Without

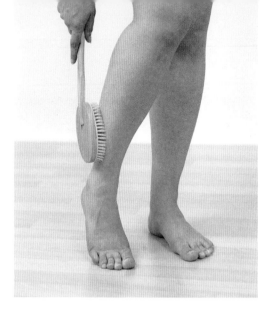

movement, the body becomes stagnant. Moving first thing in the morning will wake up your body and give you more energy throughout the day.

Dry-brush Your Body

Dry-brushing your skin will kick-start your lymphatic system, which aids in detoxification. Dry-brushing also keeps skin soft, removes dry or dead skin, and helps to maintain healthy circulation.

To dry-brush your body, you will need a soft-bristle skin brush. Starting at your feet and using upward brush strokes, work your way up your body toward your heart. Dry-brush your entire body, excluding for your face.

Take a Warm Shower or Bath Infused with Essential Oils

Most people don't have time to take a morning bath, but it's a beautiful way to start your day and set a positive energetic mood. Adding a couple of essential oils (see page 131) to your bathtub or shower in the morning will wake up your senses and invigorate your body. Essential oils such as citrus aid in boosting mood and focus.

Massage Your Face

After your shower, massage your face with a nourishing face oil, such as the Glowing Goddess Face Oil (see page 141), to protect and hydrate your skin. Rub the oil into your hands and then apply generously to your entire face and décolletage area. Using upward strokes, pay particular attention to puffy areas by pressing and releasing along the inflamed regions. Very gently massage around the eye area as well, moving the soft tissue and skin in an upward motion and taking care not to get oil in your eyes.

Drink Celery Juice Elixir

Drinking Celery Juice Elixir (see page 53) before eating food in the morning may help improve your overall health. Celery juice is nature's electrolyte. Celery is rich in sodium, magnesium, potassium, chloride, and phosphorus, all of which help to restore the body's natural electrolyte balance. Celery also balances and alkalizes the body, improves digestion, reduces inflammation, restores adrenals, improves skin, reduces water retention, and lowers bad cholesterol levels.

Enjoy a Balancing Breakfast

It is important to eat a balancing breakfast (see pages 110–113) before you start to work, teach, learn, or play. Food is our first form of medicine. Nourishing your body with foods that are balancing to your body is important in the process of self-healing. Without food, we have no fuel to burn.

Evening Routine: The Best Sleep You'll Ever Have

Sleep nourishes your body like a mother nurtures her baby. It gives you everything: strength, fertility, knowledge, contentment, happiness, and life itself. Healthy physiological, psychological, and neurological functioning all depend on you getting enough quality sleep.

We all know that sleep is a basic human need, like eating and drinking, and yet many of us still believe that we can get by on less sleep with no negative consequences. In fact, obtaining a sufficient amount of quality sleep that's in sync with your body's natural internal clock is vital for your mental and physical health. Inadequate sleep is linked to a number of conditions, including heart disease, kidney disease, high blood pressure, diabetes, stroke, obesity, and depression.

So what's the secret to waking up happier and well-rested? It's a smarter nighttime routine. What we choose to do with our evening hours directly impacts our quality of sleep, significantly influencing our mood and energy levels the next day. The truth is, most of us spend our nights

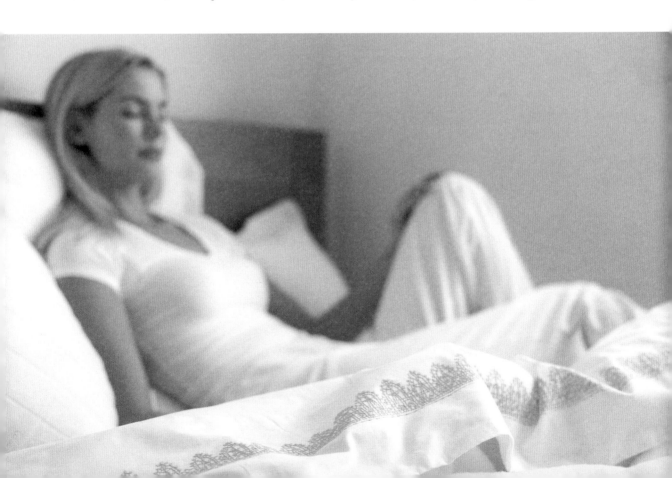

binge-watching TV shows, texting, and late-night snacking—none of which are great for catching quality sleep. The good news: Revamping your bedtime routine can be easy—and fun.

Cultivating a soothing sleep routine will help you achieve the best sleep you'll ever have. As a starting point, create a clean sleeping space, invest in comfortable bedding and keep it simple, keep the bedroom temperature low, and use nightlights if you have to get up for the bathroom during the night. Organizing your bedroom to create an at-home sleeping sanctuary is key for keeping your mind relaxed and free of stimulation in the evening hours. Try to keep your use of electronic devices to a minimum and stop using them 30 minutes before bed.

In terms of a routine, use the following practices daily to enhance your sleep, bring sacredness to your bedtime, and balance your body and mind.

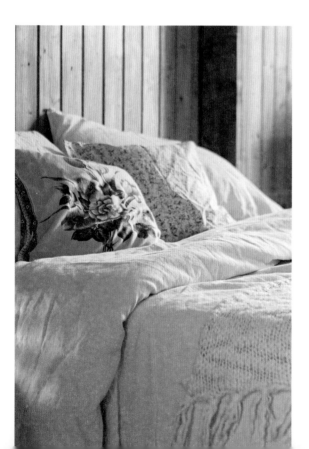

Set the Mood

Light candles and play sleep sounds to help you ease into bedtime (see page 157). Take caution, however, and make sure to blow out candles before you fall asleep. Aromatherapy and diffusing essential oils also offer a great way to create a sacred sleeping environment. Choosing a relaxing scent or blend to work naturally with your body will increase relaxation and promote restful sleep (see page 131).

Drink a Warm Adaptogenic Sleep Milk

Milk is the first thing we humans consume after birth. Drinking spiced milk is like nurturing yourself with maternal care before bed. Make drinking the Adaptogenic Sleep Milk (see page 105) an introduction to your routine, and drink it as you follow the next steps.

Give Yourself a Massage

When warm oil is absorbed into the skin, it nourishes all parts of the body, enhances circulation, and stimulates the lymphatic system. The act of self-massage (see page 134) is a nurturing ritual involving the sense of touch, an important healing tool in Ayurveda. Oiling the external body helps to ground energy and relieve stress, which is helpful for winding down to sleep.

Give Yourself a Face Mask

Paying attention to your head is a wonderful way to relax tight nerves and remove the stress of a long day. Make and apply one of the natural face masks from pages 139–140 and let the herbal infusion intoxicate and calm your senses.

Take a Relaxing Chamomile Bath

Taking time to bathe in the healing power of water can be transformative. In fact, the simple pleasure of a taking a Relaxing Chamomile Bath (see page 138) can be the perfect medicine for relaxing the body and mind after a hard day. The sensuous comfort water provides connects us back to both our bodies and the Earth's beauty.

Write in Your Journal

Sometimes our minds take control of our senses and we can't rest because our mind isn't at rest. Journaling is a practice that can help soothe your thoughts and allow your mind to rest with ease. Keep a journal or notebook by your bedside and use it to write down your thoughts, whether it's a simple reminder, such as "don't forget to buy conditioner," or a poem you're composing or deep emotional feelings that need to be let out.

Give Yourself a Reflexology Foot Massage

Reflexology involves stimulating the reflex points on your feet, hands, face, or ears to subtly impact the entire body, affecting the organs and glands. It can transport you into a state of deep relaxation where you are open to suggestions you give yourself. There are nearly 15,000 nerves in your feet alone, which is one of many reasons why foot reflexology is so calming, soothing, and effective. A simple foot-massage routine just before you go to bed can help you drift off to sleep naturally. Use an Ayurvedic massage oil such as Brahmi oil to help promote relaxation to the nerves and prevent insomnia.

To give yourself a foot massage, put 1 teaspoon of oil into the palm of your hand, rub your hands together and then massage the oil all over your

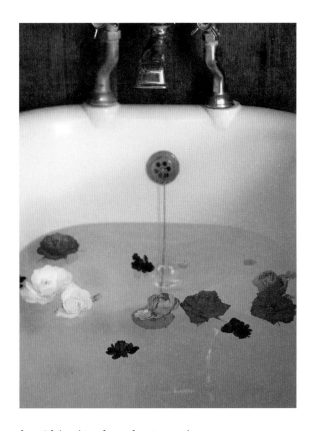

feet. (If the skin of your feet is very dry, you may want to use more oil.) Using firm pressure, slowly massage along the arch of each foot. Massage back and forth along each foot, paying particular attention to any areas that feel sore. Do this massage for at least 10 minutes.

Adapting Your Routines for Your Dosha

Cultivating inner peace takes practice and effort, especially in this busy, toxic world. You may not find it possible to do both the morning and evening routines every day. Don't worry. Having a nightly routine is important, but it's not as important as a morning routine—although this also depends on your dosha. Some doshas benefit more with a focus on the morning rather than the evening, and vice versa. Don't overwhelm yourself by trying to introduce all the suggested morning and nightly routines at once. Instead, focus on one new tool at a time and do it until it becomes a habit. With that in mind, start with the routines that are best for your dosha (see below).

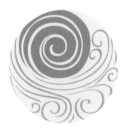

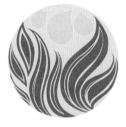

VATA People with a Vata constitution need calming, relaxing energy and, although it may feel counterintuitive, they need adequate rest. Since Vatas usually sleep sporadically and poorly, following the evening routine is very important and is more important than a morning routine. Self-massage, a warm bath, a sleep tonic (such as the Adaptogenic Sleep Milk on page 105), and a foot massage will do Vata the most benefit at night. The more Vatas can rest, the less likely they are to be imbalanced.

PITTA People with a Pitta constitution are naturally driven and ambitious, which is why keeping a morning routine is more important for them than an evening routine. Pittas need rejuvenation and slow-flowing routines. They can burn out easily and experience adrenal fatigue and lethargy if they do too much at once. Meditation, washing the face and eyes with cool water, drinking Celery Juice Elixir (see page 53), and eating a balancing breakfast will all help Pittas stay calm and cool throughout the day.

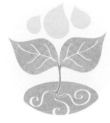

KAPHA People with a Kapha constitution tend to be sluggish and overindulge in rest, which is why an invigorating morning routine is perfect for getting them moving and maintaining a healthy balance. Rising with the sun (and by 10 a.m. at the latest) will have a positive effect on a Kapha's energy throughout the day. Drinking warm water with lemon first thing in the morning and undertaking stimulating movement like Pilates, running, cycling, or high-intensity interval training (HIIT) will help Kaphas combat sluggishness. Dry-brushing the entire body will encourage detoxification and movement of the lymph tissues (something Kaphas struggle with), and warm showers with invigorating essential oils such as citrus will keep a Kapha's energy high throughout the day. Kaphas will also enjoy the sleep routine, but they don't need it as much as the other doshas because they can usually fall asleep anywhere at any time.

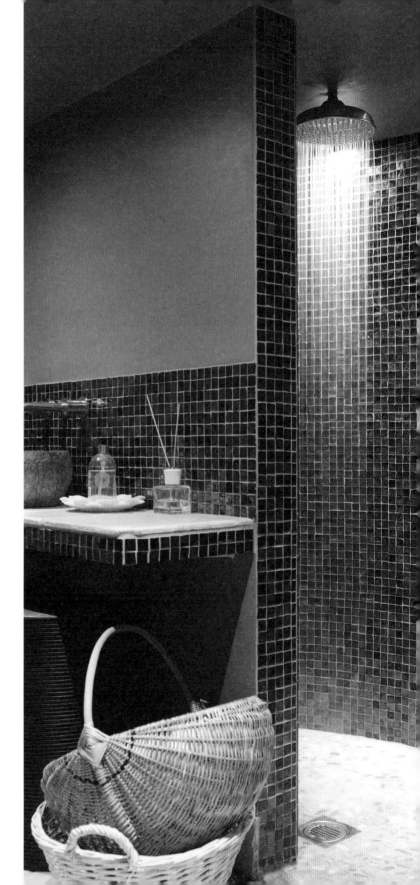

Resources: Life-enhancing Tools and Materials

The life-enhancing tools that I have provided in this section are essential to keep on hand and in your home to make your life and self-healing journey easier. These simple and accessible materials can be bought and appreciated at any time throughout your journey but they are not an essential investment in order to practice Ayurveda or heal yourself. At the time of writing this book, the brands listed below ship internationally (or have separate websites for the US and UK) unless otherwise stated.

OILS

As I've mentioned throughout this book, the quality of the oils you ingest and put on your body matters greatly. Oils you ingest should always be organic and cold pressed. Stay away from processed vegetable oils and stick to less modified oils such as olive oil.

Wonder Valley (US only: welcometowondervalley.com) makes my favorite decadent cold-pressed olive oil that can be used in most recipes.

Maharishi Ayurveda (mapi.com and maharishi.co.uk) is a premier Ayurveda brand that hosts high-quality massage oils and Ayurvedic herbs (such as triphala) and lifestyle supplements. I suggest investing in either its Vata, Pitta, or Kapha massage oil for all your self-massage needs. Alternatively, you can purchase a base oil appropriate for your dosha and add your own essential oils to it (see page 133).

The quality of essential oils you use on your body is also important. They should always be organic and without fillers. If you are buying generic essential oils cheaply, I suggest you look into the sourcing of the brand to make sure they meet the standards of a good-quality oil.

Young Living (youngliving.com/en_US and youngliving.com/en_GB–UK) has set the bar high for the way essential oils should be made with its own seed-seal process. These quality commitments are built upon three pillars: sourcing, science, and standards. Young Living is an essential oil company that I've been using since I was 14 years old. I love the quality and transparency of its products, I use them in my own recipes. Young Living carries an array of essential oils, household cleaning solutions, supplements, and body-care and baby products, all of which I highly recommend investing in. Young Living also supplies the only essential oils that I would recommend ingesting, which are called Vitality Essential Oils in the US and the Plus Oil Range in the UK.

Poppy and Someday (poppyandsomeday.com) is my recommended and favorite brand for oil-pulling oil. All its products are made in small batches, which ensures that the company pays attention to the quality of its goods. When looking for a quality oil-pulling oil, make sure that it's organic, cold-pressed, and minimally processed–if the oil contains essential oils, it is vital that the oils are food grade. There should be no fillers or unrecognizable ingredients in an oil-pulling oil since you are putting it into your mouth–the cleaner, the better.

SPICES, ADAPTOGENS, AND HERBS

Always choose organic and minimally processed spices, herbs, and adaptogens. Buying herbs in bulk will be beneficial in the long run, especially if you are excited to incorporate the tools in this book into your lifestyle. I've suggested some of my preferred suppliers below but you can also source many organic herbs in bulk from Amazon, Whole Foods, or your local boutique natural medicine shops.

Mountain Rose Herbs (mountainroseherbs.com–US/Canada only) has a wonderful wide selection of bulk herbs, spices, and other holistic DIY products. You can find organic options on the website.

Banyan Botanicals (banyanbotanicals. com–US only) is another option for Ayurvedic herbs and spices, including triphala (as well as essential oils). Its products are organic. I use them in many of my personal formulas.

I am pretty picky when it comes to the sourcing of my tonic herbs and adaptogens. The three brands I can always depend on to supply me and my clients with the absolute best and cleanest herbs are Sun Potion (sunpotion.com—also stocks triphala), Vitajing Herbs (vitajing.com), and SuperFeast (superfeast.com.au). I use all three of these brands on a daily basis to make tonics, elixirs, face masks, and mix in with food.

NATURAL SWEETENERS

Omica Organics (omicaorganics.com) creates the only liquid stevia I use and suggest to purchase. It also carries the most potent magnesium flakes you'll find on the market.

I use monk fruit sugar daily in my desserts; it scores zero on the glycemic index and is safe for diabetics. There are many different brands of monk fruit sugar available on Amazon and in health food stores.

Beekeeper's Naturals (beekeepersnaturals.com) practice sustainable beekeeping and are my trusted source for raw honey. None of their bee pollen or honey is ever heated or treated with chemicals or preservatives.

ACCESSORIES

It's not necessary to buy all these products at once, but if you feel in alignment with any of them in particular, I suggest incorporating them into your routines and rituals.

Smudge sticks and incense

Palo santo, sage, and incense have been used for centuries to protect, cleanse, and enhance rituals and sacred ceremonies. You can find smudge kits and nontoxic incense kits on Amazon and in health food stores. These kits make sweet gifts for friends and family, and you can find many beautiful homemade options on Etsy.

Candles

The type of candle you buy is important because you want the air in your home to be as clean as possible. Choose candles made from nontoxic, organic coconut wax, beeswax, or soy wax. They will intoxicate your home with beautiful scents.

Salts

SaltWorks (seasalt.com) carries organic Epsom salts in bulk. If you are planning on taking plenty of baths, I highly recommend purchasing the 50 lb (22.6 kg) bag. You can also find Epsom salts at your local pharmacy and health food store.

Tongue scrapers

A tool I can't live without—and I bet you won't be able to either once you try it—is a tongue scraper. You can order a stainless steel or copper tongue scraper on Amazon or find one at a health food store.

Skin brushes

Dry brushing (see page 150) is a must for skin health (especially for Kapha types). Karmameju (capbeauty.com/collections/karmameju) carries my favorite body and facial brushes.

Squatty Potty

Squatty Potty (squattypotty.com and squattypotty.co.uk) is a wonderful option to assist in making elimination complete. You can order fancier stools online but Squatty Potty covers everything you need. They even carry a "ghost" version that is clear so it won't be visible to guests in your bathroom.

MEDITATION

Download the Calm app (calm.com) for meditation guidance, sleep sounds, and bedtime stories. This app has changed my nightly rituals, I love listening to sleep stories about lavender fields in the south of France. It also makes for delicious dreams.

MANTRAS

If you would like to download or listen to traditional mantras, find Snatam Kaur on iTunes or online (snatamkaur.com) —her music is powerful and uplifting. To learn more about the traditional use of mantras, visit the RA MA Institute online (ramayogainstitute.com).

MY WEBSITE

My website (noellekovary.com) will give you direct access to current blog posts, videos, tutorials, free content, quizzes, products, and support for your self-healing journey. You can read more about my life, my journey toward wellness, and the little extras that have helped me and my clients heal. You will find an option to reach out to me personally and have one-on-one mentoring as well. You can find all the products I've mentioned available to order in the online store to support your self-healing journey.

You can also search my Amazon store, Noelle Kovary's Apothecary, to find my favorite products and tools: amazon.com/shop/influencer-72edccf7

There is also The Self-Healing Revolution private Facebook tribe, which you can find via my Facebook page (facebook.com/Ayurvedicalchemist), where you can share your journey and find support from a community of like-minded people and me.

Index

Acknowledgments

I owe much of my success, personal and professional, to many super humans who have created and shaped my life. To my mother, Laurette, you've imprinted my soul with a love and complex fascination for nature. Thank you for holding me close as I dove deep into the trenches of this sometimes painful journey. We have seen dark days but together our light outshines them all. To my dad, Chris, your unwavering love, support, and compassion have led me to the here and now. Thank you for teaching me to understand the subtleties in energy and how to heal through movement. To my sweet brother, Logan, your humor and charm have taught me that lightheartedness is an integral part of this journey and to always rely on the healing power of a good belly laugh. Thank you to my family for protecting me, challenging me to be better, and always keeping me grounded. Without you I wouldn't have believed that I could heal my life, let alone anyone else's.

Thank you to my partner, my best friend, the masculine to my feminine, Felipe—you have opened my world and heart to feel the power of divine love. You've showed me all that I am capable of and consistently provide me with the confidence and support to flourish.

With so much gratitude I thank Kristine Pidkameny, Carmel Edmonds, and Cindy Richards at CICO Books for believing in my vision and allowing it to come to life.

To the universe, my angels, and spirit guides, thank you for guiding me, for setting me on this path of healing, and for providing me with the vessel to experience and teach this ancient wisdom to the world.

Finally, to my teachers and all other healers, thank you for spreading consciousness, energy, and light to all those you touch. My heart and soul is with you.

Sat Nam.

Photography Credits

All photography by Stephen Conroy and © CICO Books unless otherwise stated below.

Key: a = above, b = below, c = center, ph = photographer

© RYLAND PETERS AND SMALL/ CICO BOOKS

ph Jan Baldwin: p. 16.
ph Martin Brigdale: pp. 30, 47.
ph Peter Cassidy: pp. 37ac, 53, 58b.
ph Jean Cazals: p. 58a.
ph Geoff Dann: pp. 135, 150.
ph Vanessa Davies: pp. 26a, 32.
ph Daniel Farmer: pp. 128a, 132.
ph Tara Fisher: p. 37 top.
ph Georgia Glynn-Smith: pp. 12a, 17a.
ph Catherine Gratwicke: p. 114c.
ph Winfried Heinze: pp. 42a, 130, 137.
ph Caroline Hughes: p. 37 second from bottom.
ph Erin Kunkel: pp. 28a, 28bc, 37 second from top, 37bc.

ph Adrian Lawrence: pp. 108, 109, 111 right.
ph William Lingwood: pp. 40, 128c, 138.
ph David Merewether: pp. 28ac, 142.
ph Diana Miller: p. 28c.
ph William Reavell: pp. 31, 92, 99.
ph Claire Richardson: p. 131.
ph Toby Scott: p. 29.
ph William Shaw: p. 37 bottom.
ph Debi Treloar: pp. 12c, 17c, 12b, 17b, 46, 136, 152 (www.vintagevacations. co.uk), 153.
ph Ian Wallace: p. 41.
ph Kate Whitaker: pp. 28b, 42b, 52, 83.
ph Polly Wreford: pp. 134, 151, 155 (www.coxandcox.co.uk).

© NOELLE KOVARY

pp. 98, 105, 143.
ph Benjamin Chateauvert: pp. 2, 8, 9, 26c, 35, 45, 114a, 114b, 117, 118, 128b, 139, 141, 145, 147, 149.

SHUTTERSTOCK

© fluke samed: p. 39
© Indian Food Images: p. 51
© artcasta: p. 140a
© drebha: p. 140b